Copula Additive Distributional Regression Using R

Copula additive distributional regression enables the joint modeling of multiple outcomes, an essential aspect of many real-world research problems. This book provides an accessible overview of this modeling approach, with a particular focus on its implementation in the GJRM R package, developed by the authors. The emphasis is on bivariate responses with empirical illustrations drawn from diverse fields such as health and medicine, epidemiology, economics and social sciences.

Key Features:

- Provides a comprehensive overview of joint regression modeling for multiple outcomes, with a focus on bivariate responses
- Offers a practical approach with real-world examples from various fields
- Demonstrates the implementation of all the discussed models using the GJRM package in R
- Includes supplementary resources such as data accessible through the GJRM.data package in R and additional code available on the authors' webpages

This book is designed for graduate students, researchers, practitioners and analysts who are interested in using copula additive distributional regression for the joint modeling of bivariate outcomes. The methodology is accessible to readers with a basic understanding of core statistics and probability, regression, copula modeling and R.

Chapman & Hall/CRC
The R Series

Series Editors

John M. Chambers, Department of Statistics, Stanford University, California, USA
Torsten Hothorn, Division of Biostatistics, University of Zurich, Switzerland
Duncan Temple Lang, Department of Statistics, University of California, Davis, USA
Hadley Wickham, RStudio, Boston, Massachusetts, USA

Recently Published Titles

Rasch Measurement Theory Analysis in R: Illustrations and Practical Guidance for Researchers and Practitioners
Stefanie Wind and Cheng Hua

Spatial Sampling with R
Dick R. Brus

A Criminologist's Guide to R: Crime by the Numbers
Jacob Kaplan

Analyzing US Census Data: Methods, Maps, and Models in R
Kyle Walker

ANOVA and Mixed Models: A Short Introduction Using R
Lukas Meier

Tidy Finance with R
Christoph Scheuch, Stefan Voigt, and Patrick Weiss

Deep Learning and Scientific Computing with R torch
Sigrid Keydana

Model-Based Clustering, Classification, and Density Estimation Using mclust in R
Lucca Scrucca, Chris Fraley, T. Brendan Murphy, and Adrian E. Raftery

Spatial Data Science: With Applications in R
Edzer Pebesma and Roger Bivand

Modern Data Visualization with R
Robert Kabacoff

Learn R: As a Language, Second Edition
Pedro J. Aphalo

Spatial Analysis in Geology Using R
Pedro M. Nogueira

Analyzing Baseball Data with R, Third Edition
Jim Albert, Benjamin S. Baumer and Max Marchi

Geocomputation with R, Second Edition
Robin Lovelace, Jakub Nowosad, Jannes Muenchow

Microeconometrics with R
Yves Croissant

Statistical Inference via Data Science
A ModernDive into R and the Tidyverse, Second Edition
Chester Ismay, Albert Y. Kim, and Arturo Valdivia

For more information about this series, please visit: https://www.crcpress.com/Chapman--HallCRC-The-R-Series/book-series/CRCTHERSER

Copula Additive Distributional Regression Using R

Giampiero Marra and Rosalba Radice

CRC Press
Taylor & Francis Group
Boca Raton London New York

CRC Press is an imprint of the
Taylor & Francis Group, an **informa** business

A CHAPMAN & HALL BOOK

First edition published 2026
by CRC Press
2385 NW Executive Center Drive, Suite 320, Boca Raton FL 33431

and by CRC Press
4 Park Square, Milton Park, Abingdon, Oxon, OX14 4RN

CRC Press is an imprint of Taylor & Francis Group, LLC

© 2026 Giampiero Marra and Rosalba Radice

ISBN: 978-1-032-97311-1 (hbk)
ISBN: 978-1-032-97313-5 (pbk)
ISBN: 978-1-003-59319-5 (ebk)

DOI: 10.1201/9781003593195

Typeset in LM Roman
by KnowledgeWorks Global Ltd.

*To us, as a reminder of our shared journey and vision, and to our children,
we hope you find your own path and follow it with courage and purpose.*

Contents

The Authors

Giampiero Marra is a Professor of Statistics in the Department of Statistical Science at University College London (UCL). He holds a degree in Statistics and Economics from the University of Bologna (2004) and began his career in consultancy roles in the private sector. In 2007, he completed an MSc in Statistics at UCL and successfully defended his PhD thesis at the University of Bath in November 2010. Giampiero joined UCL as a faculty member in September 2010.

Rosalba Radice is a Professor of Statistics at Bayes Business School, City St George's, University of London. After earning her PhD in Statistics from the University of Bath, she held positions as a research assistant and research fellow at the London School of Hygiene and Tropical Medicine. From 2012 to 2018, Rosalba served as Lecturer, Senior Lecturer and then Reader in Statistics at Birkbeck, University of London.

For nearly two decades, Giampiero and Rosalba have collaborated extensively to advance methodological, computational and applied statistics. Their research spans diverse areas, including penalized likelihood-based inference, copula regression and survival analysis, with impactful applications in fields such as healthcare, economics, epidemiology and the social sciences. As part of their work, they developed the GJRM package for R, which enables researchers and practitioners to implement these methods effectively while promoting transparency and reproducibility.

Preface

This book is aimed at graduate students, researchers, practitioners and data analysts who are interested in using copula additive distributional regression models to address complex real-world research problems. The primary benefit of modeling jointly bivariate or, more generally, multiple outcomes lies in the possibility of accounting for dependence between response variables, a key aspect in many applied regression analyses. For instance, when evaluating hospital performance, it is insufficient to assess in-hospital mortality without also considering length of stay, as analyzing both variables simultaneously provides a more comprehensive understanding of overall risk. Joint modeling is also relevant in causal inference, where accounting for unobserved confounding is crucial for obtaining consistent treatment effect estimates.

With a focus on bivariate responses, this book draws on empirical examples from fields such as health and medicine, epidemiology, economics and social sciences. The featured case studies showcase the advantages of the copula regression approach, demonstrating its role in fostering a more nuanced understanding of the connections between outcomes and covariates, while facilitating the derivation of model-based statistics that provide valuable insights into the underlying mechanisms driving these relationships.

The methodology described herein can handle different types of outcomes (specifically, binary, count, continuous, ordinal, survival) through several parametric distributions, supports a broad variety of dependence structures between outcomes via copulae and allows each parameter of a joint distribution to be specified as a function of an additive predictor encompassing various covariate effects. The approach is both versatile and parametric, encouraging extensive exploration of diverse functional forms, facilitating the empirical evaluation of subject matter hypotheses and enabling the straightforward computation of measures of interest. While some may view the parametric nature of the presented models as a limitation, the flexibility of the methodology can help uncover meaningful structures in the data, capturing the essence of distribution-free methods. This aligns with the view of Sir David R. Cox and others, who argued that parametric models should be more broadly utilized in empirical modeling [Reid, 1994].

The modeling framework, while sophisticated and structurally complex, does not sacrifice practical usability and interpretability of results. All the developments are incorporated into the R package GJRM [Marra and Radice, 2025a], a tool for Generalized Joint Regression Modeling that enables users to fit copula additive distributional regression models and generate intuitive numerical and visual summaries. The methodology is accessible to anyone with a basic background in core statistics and probability, regression, copula modeling and R. This book offers all the necessary material for working with GJRM in one comprehensive volume. It includes a background chapter describing the building blocks of the modeling framework and a series of chapters discussing specific models and their applications to case studies from several research areas. With an application-oriented approach, theoretical details and computational aspects are kept at a manageable level. Empirical analyses of real-world examples are designed to be easily reproducible, allowing readers to critically evaluate the models and make adjustments as needed. Although `GJRM` offers tools to assist with covariate selection, we have primarily followed a knowledge-based approach, guided by existing literature and expert opinion.

While several books discuss copula theory and distributional regression separately [Czado, 2019, Joe, 2014, Nelsen, 2006, Stasinopoulos et al., 2024, 2017, Wood, 2017], and cover diverse estimation approaches, such as boosting, Bayesian methods and likelihood-based inference, a volume that presents copula regression within a unified methodological and computational framework is lacking. Our contributions to this field are well documented through several publications [e.g., Marra and Radice, 2011, McGovern et al., 2015, Radice et al., 2016, Filippou et al., 2017, Marra and Radice, 2017, Braumoeller et al., 2018, Donat and Marra, 2018, Espasandín-Domínguez et al., 2019, Filippou et al., 2019, Marra and Radice, 2020, 2025b, van der Wurp et al., 2020, Hohberg et al., 2021, Marra and Radice, 2013a,b, 2025c]. The extensive experience gained over the years has led us to the conclusion that producing this book is the appropriate next step to advance research in copula regression and engage a broader audience. While this volume is not exhaustive, and does not aim to be, it establishes a foundation for future developments, whether by expanding the family of distributions or advancing model building tools. We are committed to continuing our research in this area and hope that future scholars will build upon and extend the class of copula regression models.

The book is organized into four parts. Part I introduces the copula additive distributional regression framework and provides a succinct overview of the `GJRM` and `GJRM.data` packages in `R`. Part II focuses on scenarios where the marginal distributions are of the same type, while Part III explores cases with mixed marginal types. Finally, Part IV demonstrates how copula regression can be applied to estimate causal treatment effects in the presence of unobserved confounding. The chapters in Parts II, III and IV follow a consistent structure: each begins with a description of a dataset that motivates the need for a particular copula model, determined primarily by the nature of the response variables of interest. This is followed by a discussion of the model and its log-likelihood, a description of the measure of interest for the chapters in Part IV, and a model fitting exercise using `GJRM`. Additional `R` code is available on the authors' websites. Readers are encouraged to start with Part I to grasp the fundamental concepts before progressing to the subsequent chapters. While some may choose to explore only those cases that align with their specific interests, reading the book comprehensively will provide a deeper understanding of the nuances of copula regression modeling.

We owe a particular debt of gratitude to the late Italo Scardovi, whom we met in 2000 while students at the University of Bologna. His *modus operandi* and keen interest in the foundational problems of inductive and deductive inference instilled in us a fervor for research in Statistical Science. We would also like to express our gratitude to Chiara Monfardini for introducing us to bivariate probit regression, our first encounter with multiple outcomes models. In 2006, our paths fortuitously crossed with Pravin Trivedi during his visit to the University of Bologna. His seminar revealed a new dimension of statistical and econometric analysis by elucidating conceptual and practical aspects of copula regression modeling, which later helped us shape our own research. We are also grateful to Simon Wood, a luminary in regression modeling and computational statistics. His mentorship inspired us to transcend conventional boundaries and foster innovation in the discipline. Finally, we would like to thank several other colleagues and friends who supported us in various ways throughout the work that led to this book. Among these are Richard Chandler, David Zimmer, Thomas Yee, Thomas Kneib, Ioannis Kosmidis, Manuel Gomes, James Nelson, Carmen María Cadarso Suárez, Francisco Gude, Irini Moustaki, Eva Cantoni, Bear F. Braumoeller, Thibault Vatter,

Thomas Nagler, Matteo Fasiolo, Francesco Donat, Elena Geminiani, Natalya Pya, Panagiota Filippou, Guy Harling, Jenifer Espasandín Domínguez, Mark E. McGovern, Małgorzata Wojtyś, Maike Hohberg, the R core team, Rob Calver and the Chapman & Hall/CRC team, the numerous people who sent us bug reports and suggested model improvements as well as new models, and the Engineering and Physical Sciences Research Council for supporting the development of some of the methods presented in this book.

Part I

The General Modeling Framework

1

Core concepts in copula regression

This chapter provides an overview of the copula additive distributional regression framework, focusing on essential elements such as copulae, marginal distributions, additive predictors and parameter estimation. Key concepts, namely effective degrees of freedom, information-based criteria, inference and residuals, are discussed to guide effective model development and evaluation. The chapter also offers an introduction to the GJRM and GJRM.data R packages, which support the implementation and illustration of the framework.

1.1 Copulae and marginal distributions

This section offers a succinct summary of the copulae and marginal distributions used in this book. For technical details on copula theory in various contexts, the reader is referred to Nelsen [2006] and Joe [2014]. For a thorough discussion of the marginal distributions, see Stasinopoulos et al. [2017].

Using the copula approach, the joint cumulative distribution function (CDF) of two outcome variables, Y_1 and Y_2, given a set of covariates, can be expressed as

$$
\begin{aligned}
\mathbb{P}(Y_1 \leq y_1, \ Y_2 \leq y_2) &= C\left(\mathbb{P}(Y_1 \leq y_1), \mathbb{P}(Y_2 \leq y_2); \theta\right) \\
&= C\left(F_1(y_1; \mu_1, \sigma_1, \nu_1), F_2(y_2; \mu_2, \sigma_2, \nu_2); \theta\right),
\end{aligned}
\tag{1.1}
$$

where $C : (0,1)^2 \to (0,1)$ is a two-place copula function with dependence parameter θ, each outcome has a CDF and a probability (density or mass) function (PDF/PMF), denoted as $F_v(y_v; \mu_v, \sigma_v, \nu_v)$ and $f_v(y_v; \mu_v, \sigma_v, \nu_v)$, for $v = 1, 2$, and the distributional parameters of these functions are specified as $g_{\mu_1}(\mu_1) = \eta_{\mu_1}(\boldsymbol{x}_{\mu_1}; \boldsymbol{\beta}_{\mu_1}), \ldots, g_{\nu_2}(\nu_2) = \eta_{\nu_2}(\boldsymbol{x}_{\nu_2}; \boldsymbol{\beta}_{\nu_2})$ and $g_{\theta}(\theta) = \eta_{\theta}(\boldsymbol{x}_{\theta}; \boldsymbol{\beta}_{\theta})$. The function $g.(\cdot)$ is a known monotonic one-to-one transformation that ensures the parameter remains within its permissible range. The additive predictor $\eta.(\boldsymbol{x}.; \boldsymbol{\beta}.) \in \mathbb{R}$ depends on a set of regressors $\boldsymbol{x}.$ and parameter vector $\boldsymbol{\beta}.$, allowing for various covariate effects as detailed in Section 1.2.

The main practical advantage of copulae is that, with knowledge of arbitrary marginal CDFs and a copula function that links them, it is possible to construct a multivariate distribution of the otherwise difficult-to-know joint CDF. Another significant benefit of the copula approach is that the selection of the marginal distributions and dependence structure can be treated as two separate but related issues, which is advantageous for model building. The copulae implemented in GJRM are listed in Table 1.1. For copulae that only support positive dependence (e.g., Clayton and Joe), counter-clockwise rotated versions can be obtained as follows: $C_{90}(u_1, u_2; \theta) = u_2 - C(1 - u_1, u_2; \theta)$, $C_{180}(u_1, u_2; \theta) = u_1 + u_2 - 1 + C(1 - u_1, 1 - u_2; \theta)$ and $C_{270}(u_1, u_2; \theta) = u_1 - C(u_1, 1 - u_2; \theta)$, where the subscript of C indicates the degree of rotation, and u_1 and u_2 are the shorthand notations for the marginal CDFs used in equation (1.1).

DOI: 10.1201/9781003593195-1

TABLE 1.1 Copulae implemented in **GJRM**, along with the corresponding parameter range for θ, relationship between Kendall's τ and θ (derived under the assumption of continuous outcomes), and range of τ. Here, u_1 and u_2 are the shorthand notations for the marginal CDFs in equation (1.1), $\Phi_2(\cdot,\cdot;\theta)$ denotes the CDF of the standard bivariate Gaussian distribution with correlation coefficient θ and $\Phi(\cdot)$ is the CDF of the standard univariate Gaussian distribution. $t_{2,\varphi}(\cdot,\cdot;\varphi,\theta)$ represents the CDF of the standard bivariate Student t-distribution with correlation θ and $\varphi \in (2,\infty)$ degrees of freedom, while $t_\varphi(\cdot)$ denotes the CDF of the standard univariate Student t-distribution with φ degrees of freedom. The Pickands dependence function of the Galambos copula is given by $A(t) = 1 - \left[t^{-\theta} + (1-t)^{-\theta}\right]^{-\frac{1}{\theta}}$. The Debye function is $D_1(\theta) = \frac{1}{\theta}\int_0^\theta \frac{t}{\exp(t)-1}dt$ and $D_2(\theta) = \int_0^1 t\log(t)(1-t)^{\frac{2(1-\theta)}{\theta}}dt$. Quantities O_1 and O_2 are defined as $O_1 = 1 + (\theta-1)(u_1+u_2)$ and $O_2 = O_1^2 - 4\theta(\theta-1)u_1 u_2$, respectively. For the Plackett copula, Kendall's τ is computed numerically. For Clayton, Galambos, Gumbel and Joe, the notation in brackets indicates the associated abbreviation and the degree of rotation, which can be 0, 90, 180 or 270.

Copula	$C(u_1, u_2; \theta)$	Range of θ	$g_\theta(\theta)$	Kendall's τ	Range of τ
Ali-Mikhail-Haq (**AMH**)	$\dfrac{u_1 u_2}{1-\theta(1-u_1)(1-u_2)}$	$[-1,1]$	$\tanh^{-1}(\theta)$	$-\dfrac{2}{3\theta^2}\left\{\theta + (1-\theta)^2 \log(1-\theta)\right\} + 1$	$[-0.1817, 1/3]$
Clayton (**C0**)	$\left(u_1^{-\theta} + u_2^{-\theta} - 1\right)^{-1/\theta}$	$(0,\infty)$	$\log(\theta)$	$\dfrac{\theta}{\theta+2}$	$(0,1]$
Farlie-Gumbel-Morgenstern (**FGM**)	$u_1 u_2 \{1 + \theta(1 - u_1)(1 - u_2)\}$	$[-1,1]$	$\tanh^{-1}(\theta)$	$\dfrac{2\theta}{9}$	$[-2/9, 2/9]$
Frank (**F**)	$-\theta^{-1}\log\left\{1 + \dfrac{(\exp\{-\theta u_1\} - 1)(\exp\{-\theta u_2\} - 1)}{(\exp\{-\theta\} - 1)}\right\}$	$\mathbb{R}\setminus\{0\}$	—	$1 - \dfrac{4}{\theta}[1 - D_1(\theta)]$	$(-1,1)\setminus\{0\}$
Galambos (**GAL0**)	$u_1 u_2 \exp\left[\left\{(-\log u_1)^{-\theta} + (-\log u_2)^{-\theta}\right\}^{-1/\theta}\right]$	$(0,\infty)$	$\log(\theta)$	$\int_0^1 \dfrac{t(1-t)}{A(t)} A''(t)dt$	$(0,1]$
Gaussian (**N**)	$\Phi_2\left(\Phi^{-1}(u_1), \Phi^{-1}(u_2); \theta\right)$	$[-1,1]$	$\tanh^{-1}(\theta)$	$\dfrac{2}{\pi}\arcsin(\theta)$	$[-1,1]$
Gumbel (**G0**)	$\exp\left[-\left\{(-\log u_1)^\theta + (-\log u_2)^\theta\right\}^{1/\theta}\right]$	$[1,\infty)$	$\log(\theta - 1)$	$1 - \dfrac{1}{\theta}$	$[0,1]$
Joe (**J0**)	$1 - \left\{(1-u_1)^\theta + (1-u_2)^\theta - (1-u_1)^\theta(1-u_2)^\theta\right\}^{1/\theta}$	$(1,\infty)$	$\log(\theta - 1)$	$1 + \dfrac{4}{\theta^2} D_2(\theta)$	$(0,1]$
Plackett (**PL**)	$\left(O_1 - \sqrt{O_2}\right)/\{2(\theta - 1)\}$	$(0,\infty)$	$\log(\theta)$	—	$(-1,1)$
Student's t (**T**)	$t_{2,\varphi}\left(t_\varphi^{-1}(u_1), t_\varphi^{-1}(u_2); \varphi, \theta\right)$	$[-1,1]$	$\tanh^{-1}(\theta)$	$\dfrac{2}{\pi}\arcsin(\theta)$	$[-1,1]$

TABLE 1.2 Definition and key properties of the main count distributions implemented in GJRM. The distributional parameters μ and σ take values in $(0, \infty)$, while $y \in \mathbb{N}_0$. Since the parameters must be positive, the transformation function $g.(\cdot) = \log(\cdot)$ is applied in all cases. $\Gamma(\cdot)$ is the gamma function, $\varpi = \sqrt{\frac{1}{\sigma^2} + \frac{2\mu}{\sigma}}$ and $\Upsilon_\hbar(\varpi) = \frac{1}{2} \int_0^\infty x^{\hbar - 1} \exp\left\{-0.5\varpi(x + x^{-1})\right\} dx$ is the modified Bessel function of the third kind. Left-truncated versions of the distributions in the table (i.e., tP, tNBI, tNBII and tPIG) at a truncation point a' are also available. These are based on the following PMF and CDF formulations: $f(y; \mu, \sigma)/\{1 - F(a'; \mu, \sigma)\}$ and $\{F(y; \mu, \sigma) - F(a'; \mu, \sigma)\}/\{1 - F(a'; \mu, \sigma)\}$.

Distribution	$f(y; \mu, \sigma)$	$\mathbb{E}(Y)$	$\mathbb{V}(Y)$
Poisson (P)	$\frac{\exp(-\mu)\mu^y}{y!}$	μ	μ
Negative binomial type I (NBI)	$\frac{\Gamma(y+1/\sigma)}{\Gamma(1/\sigma)\Gamma(y+1)} \left(\frac{\sigma\mu}{1+\sigma\mu}\right)^y \left(\frac{1}{1+\sigma\mu}\right)^{1/\sigma}$	μ	$\mu + \sigma\mu^2$
Negative binomial type II (NBII)	$\frac{\Gamma(y+\mu/\sigma)\sigma^y}{\Gamma(\mu/\sigma)\Gamma(y+1)(1+\sigma)^{y+\mu/\sigma}}$	μ	$(1+\sigma)\mu$
Poisson Inverse Gaussian (PIG)	$\left(\frac{2\varpi}{\pi}\right)^{0.5} \frac{\mu^y \exp(1/\sigma)\Upsilon_{y-0.5}(\varpi)}{(\varpi\sigma)^y y!}$	μ	$\mu + \sigma\mu^2$

A potential challenge with copula models, when one or both margins are not continuous, is the identifiability of the copula function. However, as several authors have noted [e.g., Trivedi and Zimmer, 2007, Yang et al., 2020], this issue is generally not considered a concern in a regression context with continuous covariates. This is because such regressors expand the range of $F_v(y_v; \mu_v, \sigma_v, \nu_v)$ from discrete points to a continuous interval, allowing the copula to be uniquely determined within the region defined by the possible values of $(F_1(y_1; \mu_1, \sigma_1, \nu_1), F_2(y_2; \mu_2, \sigma_2, \nu_2))$.

There are several options for specifying the marginals. For binary outcomes, $Y_v \in \{0, 1\}$, the Bernoulli distribution is a natural choice. Its PMF is $f_v(y_v; \mu_v) = \mu_v^{y_v}(1 - \mu_v)^{1-y_v}$, where $g_{\mu_v}(\mu_v) = \eta_{\mu_v}(\boldsymbol{x}_{\mu_v}; \boldsymbol{\beta}_{\mu_v})$ and $\mu_v \in (0, 1)$ represents $\mathbb{P}(Y_v = 1)$. The function $g.(\cdot)$ can be specified in three ways: $g_{\mu_v}(\mu_v) = \Phi^{-1}(\mu_v)$, the inverse of $\Phi(\cdot)$, the CDF of the standard Gaussian distribution; $g_{\mu_v}(\mu_v) = \log(\mu_v/(1 - \mu_v))$, the inverse of the standard logistic CDF; $g_{\mu_v}(\mu_v) = \log(-\log(1 - \mu_v))$, the inverse of the standard Gumbel CDF. These correspond to the probit, logit and cloglog link functions, respectively. Recall that $\mathbb{E}(Y_v) = \mu_v$ and $\mathbb{V}(Y_v) = \mu_v(1 - \mu_v)$.

For count and continuous outcomes, the possible choices are listed in Tables 1.2 and 1.3, which are parametrized according to Stasinopoulos et al. [2017]. As shown in the tables, the expectations and variances of several distributions are expressed as functions of their respective parameters. The next sections discuss the case of a survival outcome and the Tweedie distribution.

For the specific case of binary outcomes, GJRM also supports the specification of trivariate additive regression models, using the Gaussian copula [Filippou et al., 2019].

1.1.1 Survival outcome

Flexible and interpretable models for the survival function of a response variable Y, $S(y)$, can be derived from the transformation model

$$L(Y) = \eta_\mu(\boldsymbol{x}_\mu; \boldsymbol{\beta}_\mu) + \varepsilon,$$

where $L(\cdot)$ is an increasing transformation function, subject to monotonicity constraints imposed using the method discussed in Section 1.2.4, and ε is a random error specified by

TABLE 1.3 Definition and key properties of the main continuous distributions implemented in GJRM. Note that the expression for $\mathbb{E}(Y)$ and $\mathbb{V}(Y)$ for DAGUM, FISK (also known as log-logistic) and SM are indeterminate for certain values or combinations of σ and ν. If a parameter can only take positive values, the transformation function $g(\cdot) = \log(\cdot)$ is applied. For parameters constrained to the range $(0,1)$, the inverse of the CDF of the standard logistic distribution is used. In the equations, $I_B(\cdot;\cdot;\cdot)$ denotes the regularized beta function, $B(\cdot,\cdot)$ the beta function, $\Gamma(\cdot)$ the gamma function, $\gamma(\cdot,\cdot)$ the lower incomplete gamma function, $\Phi(\cdot)$ the CDF of the standard univariate Gaussian distribution and erf$(\cdot)$ the error function.

Distribution	$F(y;\mu,\sigma,\nu)$	$f(y;\mu,\sigma,\nu)$	$\mathbb{E}(Y)$	$\mathbb{V}(Y)$	Support of y / Parameter ranges
Beta (BE)	$I_B(y;\alpha_1,\alpha_2)$ $\alpha_1 = \frac{\mu(1-\sigma^2)}{\sigma^2}$ $\alpha_2 = \frac{(1-\mu)(1-\sigma^2)}{\sigma^2}$	$\frac{y^{\alpha_1-1}(1-y)^{\alpha_2-1}}{B(\alpha_1,\alpha_2)}$	μ	$\sigma^2\mu(1-\mu)$	$0 < y < 1$ $0 < \mu < 1, 0 < \sigma < 1$
Dagum (DAGUM)	$\left\{1+\left(\frac{y}{\mu}\right)^{-\sigma}\right\}^{-\nu}$	$\frac{\sigma\nu}{y}\frac{\left(\frac{y}{\mu}\right)^{\sigma\nu}}{\left\{\left(\frac{y}{\mu}\right)^{\sigma}+1\right\}^{\nu+1}}$	$-\mu\frac{\Gamma\left(-\frac{1}{\sigma}\right)\Gamma\left(\frac{1}{\sigma}+\nu\right)}{\sigma\Gamma(\nu)}$ if $\sigma > 1$	$-\mu^2\left[2\sigma\frac{\Gamma\left(-\frac{2}{\sigma}\right)\Gamma\left(\frac{2}{\sigma}+\nu\right)}{\Gamma(\nu)} - \left(\frac{\mu}{\sigma}\right)^2\left\{\frac{\Gamma\left(-\frac{1}{\sigma}\right)\Gamma\left(\frac{1}{\sigma}+\nu\right)}{\Gamma(\nu)}\right\}^2\right]$ if $\sigma > 2$	$\mu > 0, \sigma > 0, \nu > 0$
Fisk (FISK)	$\left\{1+\left(\frac{y}{\mu}\right)^{-\sigma}\right\}^{-1}$	$\frac{\sigma y^{\sigma-1}}{\mu^{\sigma}\left\{1+\left(\frac{y}{\mu}\right)^{\sigma}\right\}^2}$	$\mu\frac{\pi/\sigma}{\sin(\pi/\sigma)}$ if $\sigma > 1$	$\mu^2\left\{\frac{2\pi/\sigma}{\sin(2\pi/\sigma)} - \frac{(\pi/\sigma)^2}{\sin(\pi/\sigma)^2}\right\}$ if $\sigma > 2$	$\mu > 0, \sigma > 0$
Gamma (GA)	$\frac{1}{\Gamma\left(\frac{1}{\sigma^2}\right)}\gamma\left(\frac{1}{\sigma^2}, \frac{y}{\mu\sigma^2}\right)$	$\frac{1}{(\mu\sigma^2)^{\frac{1}{\sigma^2}}}\frac{y^{\frac{1}{\sigma^2}-1}\exp\left(-\frac{y}{\mu\sigma^2}\right)}{\Gamma\left(\frac{1}{\sigma^2}\right)}$	μ	$\mu^2\sigma^2$	$y > 0$ $\mu > 0, \sigma > 0$
Gumbel (GU)	$1-\exp\left\{-\exp\left(\frac{y-\mu}{\sigma}\right)\right\}$	$\frac{1}{\sigma}\exp\left\{\left(\frac{y-\mu}{\sigma}\right) - \exp\left(\frac{y-\mu}{\sigma}\right)\right\}$	$\mu - 0.57722\sigma$	$\frac{\pi^2\sigma^2}{6}$	$-\infty < y < \infty$ $-\infty < \mu < \infty, \sigma > 0$
Inverse Gaussian (IG)	$\Phi\left\{\frac{1}{\sqrt{y\sigma^2}}\left(\frac{y}{\mu}-1\right)\right\} + \exp\left(\frac{2}{\mu\sigma^2}\right)\Phi\left\{-\frac{1}{\sqrt{y\sigma^2}}\left(\frac{y}{\mu}+1\right)\right\}$	$\frac{1}{\sqrt{2\pi\sigma^2 y^3}}\exp\left\{-\frac{1}{2\mu^2\sigma^2 y}(y-\mu)^2\right\}$	μ	$\mu^3\sigma^2$	$y > 0$ $\mu > 0, \sigma > 0$

(*Continued.*)

TABLE 1.3 (*Continued.*)

Distribution	CDF	pdf	mean	variance	range
Log-normal (LN)	$\frac{1}{2}+\frac{1}{2}\text{erf}\left\{\frac{\log(y)-\mu}{\sigma\sqrt{2}}\right\}$	$\frac{1}{y\sigma\sqrt{2\pi}}\exp\left[-\frac{\{\log(y)-\mu\}^2}{2\sigma^2}\right]$	$\exp(\mu)\sqrt{\exp(\sigma^2)}$	$\exp(\sigma^2)\{\exp(\sigma^2)-1\}\exp(2\mu)$	$y>0$, $-\infty<\mu<\infty,\sigma>0$
Logistic (LO)	$\frac{1}{1+\exp\left(-\frac{y-\mu}{\sigma}\right)}$	$\frac{1}{\sigma}\left\{\exp\left(-\frac{y-\mu}{\sigma}\right)\right\}\left\{1+\exp\left(-\frac{y-\mu}{\sigma}\right)\right\}^{-2}$	μ	$\frac{\pi^2\sigma^2}{3}$	$-\infty<y<\infty$, $-\infty<\mu<\infty,\sigma>0$
Normal (N)	$\frac{1}{2}\left\{1+\text{erf}\left(\frac{y-\mu}{\sigma\sqrt{2}}\right)\right\}$	$\frac{1}{\sigma\sqrt{2\pi}}\exp\left\{-\frac{(y-\mu)^2}{2\sigma^2}\right\}$	μ	σ^2	$-\infty<y<\infty$, $-\infty<\mu<\infty,\sigma>0$
Reverse Gumbel (rGU)	$\exp\left\{-\exp\left(-\frac{y-\mu}{\sigma}\right)\right\}$	$\frac{1}{\sigma}\exp\left\{\left(-\frac{y-\mu}{\sigma}\right)-\exp\left(-\frac{y-\mu}{\sigma}\right)\right\}$	$\mu+0.57722\sigma$	$\frac{\pi^2\sigma^2}{6}$	$-\infty<y<\infty$, $-\infty<\mu<\infty,\sigma>0$
Singh-Maddala (SM)	$1-\left\{1+\left(\frac{y}{\mu}\right)^\sigma\right\}^{-\nu}$	$\frac{\sigma\nu y^{\sigma-1}}{\mu^\sigma\left\{1+\left(\frac{y}{\mu}\right)^\sigma\right\}^{\nu+1}}$	$\mu\frac{\Gamma\left(1+\frac{1}{\sigma}\right)\Gamma\left(-\frac{1}{\sigma}+\nu\right)}{\Gamma(\nu)}$ if $\sigma\nu>1$	$\mu^2\left\{\Gamma\left(1+\frac{2}{\sigma}\right)\Gamma(\nu)\Gamma\left(-\frac{2}{\sigma}+\nu\right)-\Gamma\left(1+\frac{1}{\sigma}\right)^2\Gamma\left(-\frac{1}{\sigma}+\nu\right)^2\right\}$ if $\sigma\nu>2$	$y>0$, $\mu>0,\sigma>0,\nu>0$
Weibull (WEI)	$1-\exp\left\{-\left(\frac{y}{\mu}\right)^\sigma\right\}$	$\frac{\sigma}{\mu}\left(\frac{y}{\mu}\right)^{\sigma-1}\exp\left\{-\left(\frac{y}{\mu}\right)^\sigma\right\}$	$\mu\Gamma\left(\frac{1}{\sigma}+1\right)$	$\mu^2\left[\Gamma\left(\frac{2}{\sigma}+1\right)-\left\{\Gamma\left(\frac{1}{\sigma}+1\right)\right\}^2\right]$	$y>0$, $\mu>0,\sigma>0$

TABLE 1.4 Definition of the survival link functions implemented in GJRM. $\Phi(\cdot)$ denotes the CDF of the standard Gaussian distribution. Note that using `-cloglog` and `-logit` leads to models with proportional hazards and proportional odds structures, respectively.

Link	$g_S(S)$	$g_S^{-1}(\eta_S)$
`-cloglog`	$\log\left\{-\log(S)\right\}$	$\exp\left\{-\exp(\eta_S)\right\}$
`-logit`	$-\log\left(\frac{S}{1-S}\right)$	$\frac{\exp(-\eta_S)}{1+\exp(-\eta_S)}$
`-probit`	$-\Phi^{-1}(S)$	$\Phi(-\eta_S)$

the standard Gaussian, logistic or Gumbel CDF. The transformation model can be written as

$$g_S\{S(y)\} = L(y) - \eta_\mu(\boldsymbol{x}_\mu; \boldsymbol{\beta}_\mu) = \eta_S(x_S; \boldsymbol{\beta}_S), \qquad (1.2)$$

where the link function $g_S(\cdot)$ is defined in Table 1.4, $L(y)$ represents the negative of the baseline survival function and $\eta_S(x_S; \boldsymbol{\beta}_S)$ is an additive predictor that depends on $x_S = \left(y, \boldsymbol{x}_\mu^\top\right)^\top$ and parameter vector $\boldsymbol{\beta}_S$.

For an accessible overview of both standard and more specialized survival models, see Royston and Lambert [2011]. For more details on the specific approach discussed here, see Marra and Radice [2020] and related works such as Cheng et al. [1995], Doksum and Gasko [1990] and Younes and Lachin [1997].

1.1.2 Tweedie distribution

If an outcome variable exhibits a substantial fraction of zero values, then the Tweedie may be a suitable choice. Applications of this distribution can be found in several research fields (see, e.g., Lee and Whitmore [1993], Jørgensen and Souza [1994], Kendall [2007], Shono [2008], Foster and Bravington [2013], Yang [2024]).

The Tweedie has the power mean-variance relationship $\mathbb{V}(Y) = \sigma\mu^\nu$, where $\mu = \mathbb{E}(Y) > 0$, $\sigma > 0$ is the scale parameter and $\nu \in \mathbb{R}$ is the shape. The implementation in GJRM covers the case where $\nu \in (1,2)$, which means that a Tweedie random variable can be represented as the sum of N independent Gamma-distributed random variables $w_1, \ldots, w_N$ with shape $-\alpha$ and scale γ, where $\alpha = (2-\nu)/(1-\nu)$, $\gamma = \sigma(\nu-1)\mu^{\nu-1}$ and N follows a Poisson distribution with rate $\omega = \mu^{2-\nu}/\sigma(2-\nu)$. The resulting density is supported on $\mathbb{R}_0^+$. The transformation functions for the distributional parameters are $g_\mu(\mu) = \log(\mu)$, $g_\sigma(\sigma) = \log(\sigma)$ and $g_\nu(\nu) = \log((\nu-1.001)/(1.999-\nu))$.

The density of the Tweedie is

$$f(y; \mu, \sigma, \nu) = a(y, \sigma, \nu) \exp\left[\frac{1}{\sigma}\{y\vartheta - \kappa(\vartheta)\}\right],$$

where

$$\vartheta = \frac{\mu^{1-\nu}}{1-\nu} \quad \text{for } \nu \neq 1 \quad \text{and} \quad \vartheta = \log\mu \quad \text{for } \nu = 1,$$

and

$$\kappa(\vartheta) = \frac{\mu^{2-\nu}}{2-\nu} \quad \text{for } \nu \neq 2 \quad \text{and} \quad \kappa(\vartheta) = \log\mu \quad \text{for } \nu = 2.$$

The quantity $a(y, \sigma, \nu)$ does not have a closed-form expression and is approximated using specially designed numerical methods [Dunn and Smyth, 2005].

The CDF of Y is defined as

$$F(y; \mu, \sigma, \nu) = \mathbb{P}\left(\sum_{i=1}^{N} w_i < y\right) = \sum_{\bar{c}=1}^{\infty} F_G\left(\sum_{i=1}^{\bar{c}} w_i < y\right) f_P(N = \bar{c}),$$

where the second equality holds due to the Law of Total Probability, F_G is equivalent to the CDF of a Gamma distribution with parameters $-\bar{c}\alpha$ and γ, while f_P is the PMF of a Poisson with rate ω. For more details, see Marra et al. [2023].

GJRM currently only permits combining a Tweedie margin with a binary outcome. Future work will expand the options to include additional types of responses.

1.2 Additive predictor

This section discusses the construction of $\eta(\boldsymbol{x}; \boldsymbol{\beta}) \in \mathbb{R}$, where its dependence on the specific distributional parameter has been omitted for simplicity. For practical purposes, it is convenient to impose an additive structure on $\eta(\boldsymbol{x}; \boldsymbol{\beta})$ which, while it limits the inclusion of all interaction terms among the covariates, still provides a great deal of flexibility and maintains good statistical properties [Wood, 2017].

Let us define

$$\eta(\boldsymbol{x}_i; \boldsymbol{\beta}) = \beta_0 + \sum_{k=1}^{K} s_k(\boldsymbol{x}_{ki}), \ \forall i = 1, \ldots, n,$$

where n is the sample size, $\beta_0 \in \mathbb{R}$ is an overall intercept, $\boldsymbol{x}_{ki}$ denotes the kth sub-vector of $\boldsymbol{x}_i$ and the K functions $s_k(\boldsymbol{x}_{ki})$ represent generic effects chosen according to the type of covariate(s) considered. Each $s_k(\boldsymbol{x}_{ki})$ can be expressed as a linear combination of J_k basis functions $b_{kj_k}(\boldsymbol{x}_{ki})$ and regression coefficients $\beta_{kj_k} \in \mathbb{R}$ (or functions of them as discussed in Section 1.2.4), i.e.

$$s_k(\boldsymbol{x}_{ki}) = \sum_{j_k=1}^{J_k} \beta_{kj_k} b_{kj_k}(\boldsymbol{x}_{ki}).$$

The vector of evaluations $\{s_k(\boldsymbol{x}_{k1}), \ldots, s_k(\boldsymbol{x}_{kn})\}^\top$ can be written as $\boldsymbol{X}_k \boldsymbol{\beta}_k$ with $\boldsymbol{\beta}_k = (\beta_{k1}, \ldots, \beta_{kJ_k})^\top$ and design matrix $X_k[i, j_k] = b_{kj_k}(\boldsymbol{x}_{ki})$. Note that the $s_k(\cdot)$ terms are subject to centering identifiability constraints.

Each $\boldsymbol{\beta}_k$ has an associated quadratic penalty $\lambda_k \boldsymbol{\beta}_k^\top \mathbf{S}_k \boldsymbol{\beta}_k$, which is required during model fitting to enforce specific properties on the kth function, such as smoothness. The smoothing parameter $\lambda_k \in [0, \infty)$ controls the trade-off between model fit and smoothness, while $\mathbf{S}_k$ depends solely on the choice of basis functions. The overall penalty is defined as $\boldsymbol{\beta}^\top \mathbf{S}_\lambda \boldsymbol{\beta}$, where $\boldsymbol{\beta} = (\beta_0, \boldsymbol{\beta}_1^\top, \ldots, \boldsymbol{\beta}_K^\top)^\top$, $\mathbf{S}_\lambda = 0 \oplus \lambda_1 \mathbf{S}_1 \oplus \cdots \oplus \lambda_K \mathbf{S}_K$, $\oplus$ denotes the direct sum operator and $\boldsymbol{\lambda} = (\lambda_1, \ldots, \lambda_K)^\top$.

The above formulation allows for various covariate effects (e.g., nonlinear, spatial). In fact, several definitions of basis functions and penalty terms are supported by GJRM, which are based on the R package mgcv by Wood [2017]. To avoid repeatedly citing the same source, readers seeking a more detailed account of the specifications discussed here and beyond should consult Wood [2017] for a thorough discussion of the $s_k(\boldsymbol{x}_{ki})$ terms as well as additional options and settings for specifying them.

1.2.1   Effects of binary and factor variables

In such cases, $s_k(\boldsymbol{x}_{ki}) = \boldsymbol{x}_{ki}^\top \boldsymbol{\beta}_k$, where the design matrix is constructed by stacking all covariate vectors $\boldsymbol{x}_{ki}$ into $\boldsymbol{X}_k$. Typically, such effects do not have penalties applied to them. However, in certain applications, this may be advisable. As an example, when dealing with a variable that has many categories but only a few observations for some of them, the parameters for such categories may be weakly identified by the data. This may lead to computational instability and a substantial increase in the variance of the parameter estimator. In these situations, a ridge penalty (obtained by setting $\mathbf{S}_k = \mathbf{I}_k$, where $\mathbf{I}_k$ is an identity matrix) can mitigate this issue. This is equivalent to assuming that the coefficients are *i.i.d.* normal random effects with unknown variance.

The specification is

```
s(x, bs = "re")
```

where x is a factor variable.

1.2.2   Nonlinear effects

These usually involve continuous covariates and can be flexibly determined from the data using the popular and computationally efficient penalized regression spline approach. This technique avoids arbitrary modeling decisions such as choosing the degrees of polynomial terms or categorizing continuous variables.

For a continuous variable x_{ki}, the design matrix $\boldsymbol{X}_k$ contains the evaluations of the J_k known spline basis functions $b_{kj_k}(x_{ki})$ for each i. To enforce smoothness, a conventional and theoretically sound choice for $\mathbf{S}_k$ is $\int \mathbf{d}_k(x_k)\mathbf{d}_k(x_k)^\top dx_k$, where the j_k^{th} element of $\mathbf{d}_k(x_k)$ is given by $\partial^2 b_{kj_k}(x_k)/\partial x_k^2$ and the integration is over the range of x_k. This approach can accommodate virtually any reasonable definition of basis functions and $\mathbf{S}_k$.

When setting up the basis functions, the type of spline, the value for J_k and, in most cases, the knots need to be specified. For one-dimensional smooth terms, the specific choice of spline basis does not usually affect the estimated smooth function, except in special cases requiring the use of less standard spline definitions. J_k is typically set to 10 (the default) as this value offers sufficient flexibility in most applications. However, analyses with larger values can be conducted to assess the sensitivity of the results to J_k. Regarding the selection of knots, they can be placed evenly across the values of the covariate or using its percentiles. For thin-plate regression splines (the default), only J_k needs to be chosen.

The smooth specification is

```
s(x, bs = "tp", k = 10)
```

where k = 10 is the number of basis functions and bs denotes the type of spline basis (thin plate regression splines in this case, although it can also be set to "cr" for cubic regression splines and "ps" for P-splines, among others).

1.2.3   Spatial effects

Geographic effects based on an area divided into distinct sub-areas (e.g., regions or districts) can be modeled using a Gaussian Markov random field smooth. This approach leverages the information from neighboring observations across different sub-areas.

Here, $s_k(\boldsymbol{x}_{ki}) = \boldsymbol{x}_{ki}^\top \boldsymbol{\beta}_k$, where $\boldsymbol{x}_{ki}$ consists of a set of area labels, $\boldsymbol{\beta}_k = (\beta_{k1}, \dots, \beta_{kR})^\top$ represents the vector of spatial effects and R denotes the total number of sub-areas.

Thus, the design matrix linking an observation i to the corresponding spatial effect is defined as

$$\boldsymbol{X}_k[i,r] = \begin{cases} 1 & \text{if the observation belongs to region } r \\ 0 & \text{otherwise} \end{cases},$$

where $r = 1, \ldots, R$. The smoothing penalty is based on the neighborhood structure of the area units, ensuring that spatially adjacent sub-areas share similar effects. Specifically,

$$\mathbf{S}_k[r,q] = \begin{cases} -1 & \text{if } r \neq q \text{ and } r \text{ is adjacent to } q \\ 0 & \text{if } r \neq q \text{ and } r \text{ is not adjacent to } q \\ N_r & \text{if } r = q \end{cases},$$

where N_r is the total number of neighbours for region r. In a stochastic interpretation, $\boldsymbol{\beta}_k$ and the neighbourhood structure can be regarded as a Gaussian Markov random field with precision matrix $\mathbf{S}_k$.

This type of smooth is invoked using

```
s(x, bs = "mrf", xt = xt)
```

where x is a factor variable representing the area labels, "mrf" specifies the Markov random field basis and xt contains a list of polygons defining the sub-area boundaries, created according to the requirements detailed in the help page for mrf in mgcv. Note that the reduced-rank version of the smooth is employed when the argument k in s() is set to a value smaller than R.

1.2.4 Nonlinear monotonic effects

A monotonically increasing estimate of $L(y)$, in equation (1.2), can be obtained using a monotonic P-spline approach. For convenience, consider the simplified notation $L(y_i) = s(y_i) = \sum_{j=1}^{J} \tilde{\beta}_j b_j(y_i)$, where the b_j terms are B-spline basis functions of at least second order, constructed over the interval $[a,b]$ with equally spaced knots, and $\tilde{\beta}_j = f_j(\beta_j)$ denotes the jth spline coefficient. A sufficient condition for $s'(y_i) \geq 0$ over $[a,b]$ is that $\tilde{\beta}_j \geq \tilde{\beta}_{j-1} \ \forall j$. This constraint can be enforced by reparametrizing the spline coefficient vector as $\tilde{\boldsymbol{\beta}} = \mathbf{f}(\boldsymbol{\beta}) = \boldsymbol{\Sigma} \{\beta_1, \exp(\beta_2), \ldots, \exp(\beta_J)\}^\top$, where $\boldsymbol{\Sigma}[\iota_1, \iota_2] = 0$ if $\iota_1 < \iota_2$ and $\boldsymbol{\Sigma}[\iota_1, \iota_2] = 1$ if $\iota_1 \geq \iota_2$, with ι_1 and ι_2 indicating the row and column indices of the matrix, respectively. The penalty term is constructed to penalize the squared differences between adjacent β_j, starting from β_2. This is achieved by defining $\mathbf{S} = \mathbf{S}^{*\top}\mathbf{S}^*$, where $\mathbf{S}^*$ is a $(J-2) \times J$ matrix consisting of zeros except that $\mathbf{S}^*[\iota, \iota+1] = -\mathbf{S}^*[\iota, \iota+2] = 1$ for $\iota = 1, \ldots, J-2$.

The specification is

```
s(y, bs = "mpi")
```

where "mpi" refers to the monotonic increasing P-spline smooth.

1.2.5 Smooth interactions

Interaction effects between two or more covariates can be modeled using a full tensor product smooth (te), a tensor product interaction (ti), if the related main effects are included separately in the model, or an isotropic (thin-plate regression spline) smooth (s). Options te and ti are particularly useful when the covariates are measured in different units. However, for well-scaled covariates, an isotropic smooth typically performs better.

A tensor product smooth is created by combining the model and penalty matrices of the marginal bases to form a single model matrix, while retaining multiple penalties, one for each marginal basis. In contrast, constructing a thin-plate regression spline in more than one dimension results in a single model penalty. The use of `ti` more closely resembles the traditional method of including interaction terms in a model.

For two continuous variables `x1` and `x2`, such smooths can be specified using terms like

```
te(x1, x2)
ti(x1) + ti(x2) + ti(x1, x2)
s(x1, x2)
```

In addition, interactions involving numeric and factor variables can be specified using the `by` argument, which produces a varying coefficient model in the case of numeric variables, and a smooth estimate for each level in the case of factor variables.

1.3   Parameter estimation

Having discussed the construction of an arbitrary η in Section 1.2, it is now possible to define some key quantities related to the model additive predictors. Specifically, $\beta = (\beta_{\mu_1}^\top, \beta_{\mu_2}^\top, \ldots, \beta_\theta^\top)^\top$ represents the overall parameter vector for the coefficients of all the additive predictors of the model. Similarly, $\mathbf{S}_\lambda = \mathbf{S}_{\lambda_{\mu_1}} \oplus \mathbf{S}_{\lambda_{\mu_2}} \oplus \cdots \oplus \mathbf{S}_{\lambda_\theta}$ corresponds to the overall block-diagonal penalty associated with β, and $\lambda = (\lambda_{\mu_1}^\top, \lambda_{\mu_2}^\top, \ldots, \lambda_\theta^\top)^\top$ collects all the smoothing parameters. The parameter estimator $\hat{\beta}$ is obtained using a penalized maximum likelihood estimation method, as detailed below.

Due to the flexibility allowed by the copula additive distributional regression framework in specifying covariate effects, the model log-likelihood $\ell(\beta)$ is augmented by an overall quadratic penalty. Specifically,

$$\ell_p(\beta) = \ell(\beta) - \frac{1}{2}\beta^\top \mathbf{S}_\lambda \beta, \tag{1.3}$$

where $\ell(\beta)$ is defined explicitly for each case discussed in the subsequent chapters. Estimation of β and λ is carried out via the efficient and stable penalized likelihood-based approach described in the next two sections.

1.3.1   Estimation of β

At iteration *it*, for a given parameter vector $\beta^{[it]}$ and holding the smoothing parameters fixed at $\lambda^{[it]}$ or $\hat{\lambda}$, an update for β is found by solving

$$\beta^{[it+1]} = \beta^{[it]} + \underbrace{\underset{e:\|e\|\leq\Delta^{[it]}}{\operatorname{argmin}} \; \breve{\ell}_p(\beta^{[it]})}_{:=e^{[it+1]}}, \tag{1.4}$$

$$\breve{\ell}_p(\beta^{[it]}) := -\{\ell_p(\beta^{[it]}) + e^\top g_p^{[it]} + \frac{1}{2}e^\top H_p^{[it]}e\},$$

where $\|\cdot\|$ is the Euclidean norm and $\Delta^{[it]}$ is the radius of the trust region, which is adjusted throughout the iterations. The penalized score vector and penalized Hessian matrix are given by $g_p^{[it]} = g^{[it]} - \mathbf{S}_{\hat{\lambda}}\beta^{[it]}$ and $H_p^{[it]} = H^{[it]} - \mathbf{S}_{\hat{\lambda}}$, respectively, where $g^{[it]}$ is defined as

$$\left(\left. \frac{\partial \ell(\beta)}{\partial \beta_{\mu_1}} \right|^{\top}_{\beta_{\mu_1} = \beta_{\mu_1}^{[it]}}, \ldots, \left. \frac{\partial \ell(\beta)}{\partial \beta_{\theta}} \right|^{\top}_{\beta_{\theta} = \beta_{\theta}^{[it]}} \right)^{\top}$$

and $H^{[it]}$ as

$$\left. \frac{\partial^2 \ell(\beta)}{\partial \beta_l \partial \beta_m^{\top}} \right|_{\beta_l = \beta_l^{[it]}, \beta_m = \beta_m^{[it]}}, \quad l, m = \mu_1, \mu_2, \ldots, \theta.$$

At each iteration, the minimization of (1.4) uses a quadratic approximation of $\ell_p(\beta^{[it]})$ to determine the best $e^{[it+1]}$ within the ball centered at $\beta^{[it]}$ with radius $\Delta^{[it]}$.

Trust region and classical line search methods employ a quadratic model of the objective function to generate steps between iterations. Line search approaches find a search direction and then determine a suitable step length along that direction, whereas trust region techniques search for the step that minimizes the objective function within a predefined region around the current iterate. If a function exhibits, for example, long plateaus and the current iterate $\beta^{[it]}$ lies in such a region, line search procedures may search the next step $\beta^{[it+1]}$ far from the current iterate, reducing the efficiency of the algorithm. Moreover, evaluating the objective function may lead to indefinite values, causing the algorithm to fail. In contrast, trust region methods define a maximum distance before evaluating the objective function, ensuring that the new iterate is not too far from the current one. If the evaluation of $\breve{\ell}_p$ is indefinite, the step $e^{[it+1]}$ is not accepted. If the candidate step does not sufficiently improve the function or results in a non-definite evaluation of $\breve{\ell}_p$, the trust region shrinks and the algorithm returns to the previous step. If the improvement is significant, then the trust region expands in the next iteration.

Since the implementation of the models in GJRM is mainly based on the analytical score and Hessian of $\ell_p(\beta)$, the algorithm converges super-linearly to a point satisfying the second-order sufficient conditions; see Nocedal and Wright [2006, Chapter 4] for more details.

1.3.2 Estimation of λ

To discuss the criterion adopted for automatic multiple smoothing parameter estimation, $\hat{\beta}$ has to be expressed in terms of the score and Hessian. A first-order Taylor expansion of $g_p^{[it+1]}$ around $\beta^{[it]}$ yields $\mathbf{0} = g_p^{[it+1]} \approx g_p^{[it]} + \left(\beta^{[it+1]} - \beta^{[it]} \right) H_p^{[it]}$, which, after some manipulation, leads to $\beta^{[it+1]} = \left(-H_p^{[it]} \right)^{-1} \sqrt{-H^{[it]}} \mathbf{M}^{[it]}$, where $\mathbf{M}^{[it]} = \mu_{\mathbf{M}}^{[it]} + \epsilon^{[it]}$, $\mu_{\mathbf{M}}^{[it]} = \sqrt{-H^{[it]}} \beta^{[it]}$ and $\epsilon^{[it]} = \sqrt{-H^{[it]}}^{-1} g^{[it]}$. From likelihood theory, $\epsilon \sim \mathcal{N}(\mathbf{0}, \mathbf{I}_{\psi})$, $\mathbf{M} \sim \mathcal{N}(\mu_{\mathbf{M}}, \mathbf{I}_{\psi})$, where $\mathbf{I}_{\psi}$ is an identity matrix of dimension $\psi = \dim(\beta)$, $\mu_{\mathbf{M}} = \sqrt{-H} \beta^{true}$ and β^{true} is the true parameter vector. The predicted value vector for $\mathbf{M}$ is $\hat{\mu}_{\mathbf{M}} = \sqrt{-H} \hat{\beta} = \mathbf{A}\mathbf{M}$, where $\mathbf{A} = \sqrt{-H} (-H_p)^{-1} \sqrt{-H}$.

To calibrate the trade-off between fit and parsimony, λ is determined by minimizing

$$\mathbb{E}\left(\|\mu_{\mathbf{M}} - \hat{\mu}_{\mathbf{M}}\|^2 \right) = \mathbb{E}\left(\|\mathbf{M} - \mathbf{A}\mathbf{M}\|^2 \right) - Wn + 2\mathrm{tr}(\mathbf{A}), \tag{1.5}$$

where W is the total number of distributional model parameters. Note that (1.5) depends on λ through $\mathbf{A}$. In practice, an estimate of (1.5) is required, which is

$$\widehat{\|\mu_{\mathbf{M}} - \hat{\mu}_{\mathbf{M}}\|^2} = \|\mathbf{M} - \mathbf{A}\mathbf{M}\|^2 - Wn + 2\mathrm{tr}(\mathbf{A}). \tag{1.6}$$

Therefore, for a given $\boldsymbol{\lambda}^{[it]}$, while holding $\boldsymbol{\beta}^{[it+1]}$ fixed, the following problem is solved

$$\boldsymbol{\lambda}^{[it+1]} = \arg \min_{\boldsymbol{\lambda}} \|\mathbf{M}^{[it+1]} - \mathbf{A}^{[it+1]}\mathbf{M}^{[it+1]}\|^2 - Wn + 2\mathrm{tr}(\mathbf{A}^{[it+1]}), \qquad (1.7)$$

using the stable and efficient computational routine of Wood [2017, Section 6.5.1]. Basing smoothing parameter estimation on $\mathbf{M}$ and $\mathbf{A}$, which use $\boldsymbol{g}$ and $\boldsymbol{H}$ in their aggregate forms instead of the n components that make them up, enhances the stability, efficiency and modularity of the approach [Marra et al., 2017]. Additionally, the score and Hessian, required to set up the quantities in (1.7), are obtained as a byproduct of the estimation step for $\boldsymbol{\beta}$, thereby reducing the computational effort required to solve the optimization problem.

The steps for estimating $\boldsymbol{\beta}$ and $\boldsymbol{\lambda}$ are iterated until $|\ell(\boldsymbol{\beta}^{[it+1]}) - \ell(\boldsymbol{\beta}^{[it]})| / (0.1 + |\ell(\boldsymbol{\beta}^{[it+1]})|) < 1e - 07$ is satisfied.

Starting values are obtained by fitting univariate regression models using `mgcv::gam()`, `GJRM::gamlss()` or a combination of both, and by calculating the empirical correlation between the residuals of these regressions.

1.4   Effective degrees of freedom

The number of parameters in an unpenalized model is denoted by ψ. In a penalized model, the number of 'effective' parameters is given by the effective degrees of freedom, $edf = \mathrm{tr}(\mathbf{A})$, which can also be expressed as $\psi - \mathrm{tr}\left\{(-\boldsymbol{H} + \mathbf{S}_{\boldsymbol{\lambda}})^{-1}\mathbf{S}_{\boldsymbol{\lambda}}\right\}$. From this expression, it is clear that if $\boldsymbol{\lambda} \to \mathbf{0}$, then $\mathrm{tr}(\mathbf{A}) \to \psi$, and if $\boldsymbol{\lambda} \to \infty$, then $\mathrm{tr}(\mathbf{A}) \to \psi - \zeta$, where ζ is the total number of parameters subject to penalization. When $\mathbf{0} < \boldsymbol{\lambda} < \infty$, the edf falls within the range $[\psi - \zeta, \psi]$. The edf of a single smooth or penalized component is the sum of the corresponding trace elements.

1.5   Information-based criteria

The Akaike and Bayesian information criteria [Schwarz, 1978, Akaike, 1998] for a model with the number of parameters given by the edf are defined as AIC $= -2\ell(\hat{\boldsymbol{\beta}}) + 2edf$ and BIC $= -2\ell(\hat{\boldsymbol{\beta}}) + \log(n)edf$. Note that, within an additive constant, the first term on the right hand side of (1.6) is a quadratic approximation of $-2\ell(\hat{\boldsymbol{\beta}})$, making the overall equation approximately equivalent to the AIC with edf as the number of parameters.

Approaches such as the Clarke and Vuong tests can also be employed, particularly when comparing non-nested models [Vuong, 1989, Clarke, 2007]. The Clarke test is a distribution-free method used to determine whether one of two models consistently provides a better fit for individual observations. Under the null hypothesis of equivalence, the number of positive differences between the log-likelihood contributions of two models follows a binomial distribution with parameters n and 0.5. The Vuong test, on the other hand, compares two competing models by examining the difference in their log-likelihoods, standardized by the associated standard error, resulting in a statistic that follows a standard normal distribution under the null. Both tests adjust for the edfs of the models.

1.6 Inference

The construction of 'confidence' intervals is based on the Bayesian result detailed in Wood [2017, Section 6.10] for models fitted via penalized log-likelihoods of the general form (1.3). This is $\boldsymbol{\beta} \overset{.}{\sim} \mathcal{N}(\hat{\boldsymbol{\beta}}, \mathbf{V}_{\boldsymbol{\beta}})$, where $\mathbf{V}_{\boldsymbol{\beta}} = (-\hat{\boldsymbol{H}}_p)^{-1}$. Such an approach follows the notion that penalization in estimation assumes that wiggly models are less likely than smoother ones, which translates into the prior specification $f_{\boldsymbol{\beta}} \propto \exp\left\{-\boldsymbol{\beta}^{\top}\mathbf{S}_{\boldsymbol{\lambda}}\boldsymbol{\beta}/2\right\}$. Note that $\mathbf{V}_{\boldsymbol{\beta}}$ has good frequentist properties because it accounts for both sampling variability and smoothing bias. The additive predictor of a survival equation is nonlinear in the related model parameters (see Section 1.2.4). Here, to facilitate the computation of intervals, the distribution of the transformed coefficient vector, on which all the model terms depend linearly, is employed (see Marra and Radice [2020] for details).

Intervals for linear functions of the model coefficients, such as smooth terms, are easily constructed using the aforementioned result. Recall that smooth components are subject to centering identifiability constraints. In this regard, consider the case of a smooth function of a continuous covariate. When *edf* is equal to 1 (implying that the smooth is estimated as a straight line), there is no uncertainty at zero, a feature that is reflected in the intervals.

For nonlinear functions of the model coefficients (e.g., joint and conditional probabilities, θ, τ), intervals can be conveniently determined by posterior simulation as follows:

- Draw n_{sim} random vectors $\breve{\boldsymbol{\beta}}_1, \ldots, \breve{\boldsymbol{\beta}}_{n_{sim}}$ from $\mathcal{N}(\hat{\boldsymbol{\beta}}, \mathbf{V}_{\boldsymbol{\beta}})$.
- Obtain n_{sim} realizations of the function of interest. For instance, consider $\theta_i = \tanh\{\eta_{\theta}(\boldsymbol{x}_{i\theta}; \boldsymbol{\beta}_{\theta})\}$, the dependence parameter of the Gaussian copula specified as a function of covariate effects. Here, $\boldsymbol{\theta}_i^{sim} = (\theta_{i1}, \theta_{i2}, \ldots, \theta_{in_{sim}})^{\top}, \forall i = 1, \ldots, n$, is obtained using $\breve{\boldsymbol{\beta}}_{\theta 1}, \ldots, \breve{\boldsymbol{\beta}}_{\theta n_{sim}}$, extracted from the overall coefficient simulated vectors obtained in the previous step.
- For each $\boldsymbol{\theta}_i^{sim}$, calculate the lower $\varsigma/2$ and upper $1 - \varsigma/2$ quantiles.

The parameter ς is typically set to 0.05, while a value of n_{sim} equal to 100 usually produces representative results, although it can be increased for more precision. Note that the distribution of nonlinear functions of the model parameters need not be symmetric. Furthermore, unless a seed is set before executing the above steps, the procedure will usually produce slightly different intervals each time it is run; increasing n_{sim} mitigates this variability. The `n.sim` argument in several post-estimation functions provides control over this aspect.

The *p*-values for the terms in the model are obtained using the results in Wood [2017, Section 6.12], to which the reader is referred to for full details.

1.7 Residuals

`GJRM` implements two main definitions of residuals. For simplicity, the subscript indicating the specific margin to which the residuals apply has been omitted.

Normalized quantile residuals. These are appropriate for continuous outcomes and are given by $\Phi^{-1}\left\{F(y_i; \hat{\mu}_i, \hat{\sigma}_i, \hat{\nu}_i)\right\}$. Under correct model specification, the residuals follow a standard Gaussian distribution, which can be assessed by inspecting the corresponding normal Q–Q plot. For the Tweedie distribution, to account for the probability mass at zero, residuals corresponding to outcome values equal to 0 are obtained by sampling uniform variates with bounds given by 0 and the probabilities associated with these observations [Dunn and Smyth, 1996]. There is also the option of producing reference bands for the Q–Q plots, using the approach discussed by Augustin et al. [2012].

Randomized normalized quantile residuals. These are used for count outcomes and are defined as $\Phi^{-1}(\xi_i)$, where ξ_i is a random value from the uniform distribution on $[F(y_i - 1; \hat{\mu}_i, \hat{\sigma}_i, \hat{\nu}_i), F(y_i; \hat{\mu}_i, \hat{\sigma}_i, \hat{\nu}_i)]$. In practice, $F(y_i - 1; \hat{\mu}_i, \hat{\sigma}_i, \hat{\nu}_i)$ is replaced with $F(y_i; \hat{\mu}_i, \hat{\sigma}_i, \hat{\nu}_i) - f(y_i; \hat{\mu}_i, \hat{\sigma}_i, \hat{\nu}_i)$. This is particularly relevant when $y_i = 0$, in which case $F(-1)$ is set to 0. This construction allows count distributions to be treated as continuous, enabling Q–Q plots of residuals to be inspected similarly to the continuous outcome case.

GJRM does not currently include versions of residuals for cases where the outcomes are neither count nor continuous, and future work will look into addressing this gap.

1.8   Model building

In copula regression, the model building process can be streamlined by recognizing that selecting the marginal distributions and the copula function are distinct but related tasks. Using this fact, marginal distributions may be chosen first, using residual analysis and convergence checks. If several distributions appear to fit the data well, considerations of parsimony and information-based criteria can help guide the final selections. Once the marginals are determined, the next step is to select an appropriate dependence structure, starting with the Gaussian copula, a classical choice for modeling both positive and negative correlations. Depending on the sign of the observed dependence, alternative copulae can then be assessed using, for example, information-based criteria such as the Clarke and Vuong tests.

Covariate selection can be supported by tools such as shrinkage smoothers and p-values. However, this book primarily adopts a knowledge-based approach, drawing on previous literature and expert opinion.

1.9   The GJRM R package

The GJRM package is available from the Comprehensive R Archive Network (CRAN) at https://CRAN.R-project.org/package=GJRM. The main function is gjrm() which can be called using the following syntax:

```
gjrm(formula, data = list(), margins, copula = "N", model, cens1 = NULL,
     cens2 = NULL, ub.t1 = NULL, ub.t2 = NULL, uni.fit = FALSE, ...)
```

where

- formula is a list of at least two (or at least three, for trivariate binary models) formulae specified following the syntax of mgcv::gam(). Additional equations can be included depending on the number of distributional parameters in the copula additive distributional regression model. Consider, for example, a Clayton model with NBI and DAGUM margins, where each parameter of the joint distribution is specified as a function of a common additive predictor, which includes a linear effect of the binary covariate `x1` and a nonlinear effect of the continuous covariate `x2`. In this case, $C\left(F_1(y_1; \mu_1, \sigma_1), F_2(y_2; \mu_2, \sigma_2, \nu_2); \theta\right)$, where $\log(\mu_v) = \beta_{0\mu_v} + \beta_{1\mu_v}x_1 + s_{\mu_v}(x_2)$ and $\log(\sigma_v) = \beta_{0\sigma_v} + \beta_{1\sigma_v}x_1 + s_{\sigma_v}(x_2)$, for $v = 1, 2$, $\log(\nu_2) = \beta_{0\nu_2} + \beta_{1\nu_2}x_1 + s_{\nu_2}(x_2)$ and $\log(\theta) = \beta_{0\theta} + \beta_{1\theta}x_1 + s_\theta(x_2)$. The related `formula` list would be

```
eq1 <- y1 ~ x1 + s(x2)  # mu1
eq2 <- y2 ~ x1 + s(x2)  # mu2
eq3 <-    ~ x1 + s(x2)  # sigma1
eq4 <-    ~ x1 + s(x2)  # sigma2
eq5 <-    ~ x1 + s(x2)  # nu2
eq6 <-    ~ x1 + s(x2)  # theta

fl <- list(eq1, eq2, eq3, eq4, eq5, eq6)
```

- `data` is a data frame;

- `margins` is a character vector that specifies distributions, link functions or a combination of both. For a binary outcome, the default distribution is the Bernoulli, with `probit`, `logit` or `cloglog` as the link function. For an ordinal response, the available choices are the probit and logit link functions (`ord.probit` and `ord.logit`). For count, continuous and survival outcomes, the possible options are listed in the first columns of Tables 1.2, 1.3 and 1.4;

- `copula` can be set to any of the values listed in brackets next to the copula names in Table 1.1;

- `model` can be set to "B" (bivariate model), "BSS" (bivariate model with non-random sample selection), "BPO" (bivariate probit model with partial observability), "BPOO" (bivariate probit model with partial observability and $\theta = 0$), "T" (trivariate binary model), "TSS" (trivariate binary model with non-random double sample selection) and "TESS" (trivariate binary model with endogeneity and non-random sample selection);

- `cens1` and `cens2` are censoring indicators for the survival responses. For right-censored outcomes, each can be equal to 1 if the event occurred and 0 otherwise. If there are multiple censoring mechanisms, these have to be specified as factor variables with four possible categories: `I` for interval, `L` for left, `R` for right and `U` for uncensored;

- `ub.t1` and `ub.t2` are used only for interval-censored responses and represent the variable names of the upper bounds;

- if `uni.fit = TRUE` then univariate distributional regression models are internally fitted using `GJRM::gamlss()` to obtain better-calibrated starting values, although this may come at an increased computational cost. This also provides the marginal fits required to compute joint probabilities under the assumption of independence of the margins.

The following are some post-estimation functions available in `GJRM`:

- `conv.check()` provides convergence information for the fitted model. The maximum absolute value of the gradient should be close to 0, and the observed information matrix should be positive definite. Slight differences in convergence results may occur when running models on different computers or `R` versions, often due to variations in machine precision and internal software changes;

- `clarke.test()` and `vuong.test()` implement the procedures discussed in Section 1.5;

- `res.check()` produces normal Q–Q plot(s) based on the residuals described in Section 1.7;

- `marg.mv()` computes the means and variances of the marginal distributions implemented in the package;

- `cond.mv()` implements the conditional means and variances specific to the copula models covered in the book;

- `copula.prob()` computes joint and conditional probabilities from a fitted model;

- The standard R functions `summary()`, `plot()`, `AIC()` and `BIC()` can be employed as usual.

1.10   The `GJRM.data` R package

The `GJRM.data` package is available from the Comprehensive R Archive Network at https://CRAN.R-project.org/package=GJRM.data and includes the datasets used throughout the book. These originate from various fields and address challenges related to dependent bivariate outcomes, where the copula regression modeling framework is essential for uncovering valuable patterns in the data.

The following provides a brief summary of the datasets.

- Blood pressure in children (`bpc`)

    - Source: Solomon-Moore et al. [2020].

    - Aim: Joint modeling of systolic and diastolic blood pressures in 11-year-old children as functions of additive predictors based on gender, body mass index, physical activity and sedentary behavior.

- Medical expenditure panel survey (`meps`)

    - Source: Agency for Healthcare Research and Quality, U.S. Department of Health and Human Services.

    - Aims:

        * Joint modeling of number of doctor and non-doctor health visits as functions of additive predictors based on individual-level characteristics such as body mass index, income and age.

        * Simultaneous modeling of perceived general and mental health as functions of covariate effects based on individual-level features.

        * Joint modeling of the number and cost of physician visits based on patient characteristics.

- Age-related eye disease (`areds`)

    - Source: Multicenter clinical trial on age-related macular degeneration (AMD) [AREDS Group, 1999].

    - Aim: Joint modeling of progression times to late AMD in the left and right eyes as functions of covariate effects based on age, a genetic variant and baseline severity score.

- Civil war onset (`war`)
  - Source: Fearon and Laitin [2003].
  - Aim: Analysis of the determinants of civil war onset while accounting for partial observability.

- Adverse birth study (`infants`)
  - Source: North Carolina State Center for Health Statistics.
  - Aim: Joint modeling of low birth weight and preterm birth as functions of geographic and covariate effects based on maternal characteristics.

- Happiness and economic prosperity (`happy`):
  - Source: United Nations Sustainable Development Solutions Network, 2019 World Happiness Report.
  - Aim: Simultaneous modeling of happiness score and economic performance as functions of covariate effects based on healthy life expectancy and social support, among others.

- HIV status and CD4 counts (`cd4`)
  - Source: Fictitious data designed to replicate the characteristics and patterns observed in the Africa Centre Demographic Information System for women.
  - Aim: Joint modeling of HIV status and CD4 count measurements as functions of additive predictors based on variables such as age, marital status and education.

- Hospital length of stay and mortality (`hospital`)
  - Source: Lewis Gale Medical Center (2014) [Azadeh-Fard et al., 2016].
  - Aims: Joint modeling of length of stay and death as functions of covariate effects based on various individual-level health indicators.

- Illinois reemployment bonus experiment (`hie`)
  - Source: The Illinois Unemployment Incentive Experiments [Woodbury and Spiegelman, 1987].
  - Aims:
    * Estimation of the causal effect of a cash bonus on the probability of being employed, accounting for both observed and unobserved confounders.
    * Estimation of the causal effect of a cash bonus on unemployment duration, controlling for both observed and unobserved confounders.

- HIV population study (`hiv`)
  - Source: Synthetic data replicating the structure and statistical properties of the 2007 Demographic and Health Surveys.
  - Aim: Estimation of HIV prevalence adjusting for non-random participation in testing.

For more details on each dataset, the reader is referred to the corresponding help file, accessible with `?dataframe_name`.

Part II

Same Type of Marginals

2

Continuous outcomes

Copulae originated in probability theory, with Sklar's theorem playing a fundamental role in their development. Following Sklar's work, copulae gained considerable attention in the scientific community, particularly from the 1970s onward, primarily in the fields of finance and actuarial science. Since then, copula models have become increasingly popular across various disciplines, with researchers exploring their applications with different types of marginals and regression structures. Copula models with continuous margins represent the most classic case in multivariate response modeling, with applications in several areas such as insurance [Frees and Valdez, 1998, Frees and Wang, 2005], finance [Cherubini et al., 2004, Pitt et al., 2006], marketing [Danaher and Smith, 2011], medicine [Yin and Yuan, 2009, Hashizume et al., 2022] and environmental research [Bhatti and Do, 2019].

This chapter introduces the copula additive distributional regression approach developed by Marra and Radice [2017]. The model is applied to children data with a focus on the joint modeling of systolic and diastolic blood pressures, while accounting for individual-level risk factors. Various model-based measures are explored to enhance the understanding of blood pressure patterns in children.

2.1 Blood pressure in children

Elevated blood pressure in children is a significant risk factor for the development of cardiovascular disease in adulthood. This study focuses on 11-year-old children and examines how systolic and diastolic blood pressure levels (sbp and dbp) are influenced by gender, body mass index (bmi), moderate to vigorous physical activity (mvpa) and sedentary behavior (sed), measured in minutes per day via accelerometers.

Blood pressure levels are key indicators of cardiovascular health, and modeling them jointly and as functions of the aforementioned individual-level characteristics offers a more comprehensive assessment of blood pressure regulation. The insights gained from the copula regression approach can help inform the development of preventive health strategies to address cardiovascular diseases.

The dataset used in this study is a subsample from Solomon-Moore et al. [2020], comprising 1,052 observations.

2.2 Model

Let (Y_1, Y_2) be a pair of continuous random variables, and let their joint CDF be expressed as

$$\mathbb{P}(Y_1 \leq y_1,\ Y_2 \leq y_2) = C(F_1(y_1; \mu_1, \sigma_1, \nu_1), F_2(y_2; \mu_2, \sigma_2, \nu_2); \theta), \qquad (2.1)$$

where $C(\cdot, \cdot; \theta)$ is a copula function, $F_j(y_j; \mu_j, \sigma_j, \nu_j)$ is the jth marginal CDF, for $j = 1, 2$, and the distributional parameters are modeled as $g_{\mu_j}(\mu_j) = \eta_{\mu_j}(\boldsymbol{x}_{\mu_j}; \boldsymbol{\beta}_{\mu_j})$, $g_{\sigma_j}(\sigma_j) = \eta_{\sigma_j}(\boldsymbol{x}_{\sigma_j}; \boldsymbol{\beta}_{\sigma_j})$, $g_{\nu_j}(\nu_j) = \eta_{\nu_j}(\boldsymbol{x}_{\nu_j}; \boldsymbol{\beta}_{\nu_j})$ and $g_\theta(\theta) = \eta_\theta(\boldsymbol{x}_\theta; \boldsymbol{\beta}_\theta)$. Any combination of distributions from Table 1.3 can be adopted. However, since sbp and dbp cannot take negative values, only distributions with positive support are considered in the case study.

The joint PDF is given by

$$c(F_1(y_1; \mu_1, \sigma_1, \nu_1), F_2(y_2; \mu_2, \sigma_2, \nu_2); \theta) f_1(y_1; \mu_1, \sigma_1, \nu_1) f_2(y_2; \mu_2, \sigma_2, \nu_2), \qquad (2.2)$$

where the copula density $c(\cdot, \cdot; \theta)$ is defined as

$$\frac{\partial^2 C(F_1(y_1; \mu_1, \sigma_1, \nu_1), F_2(y_2; \mu_2, \sigma_2, \nu_2); \theta)}{\partial F_1(y_1; \mu_1, \sigma_1, \nu_1) \partial F_2(y_2; \mu_2, \sigma_2, \nu_2)},$$

and $f_j(y_j; \mu_j, \sigma_j, \nu_j)$ is the PDF of Y_j.

2.3 Log-likelihood

Using equation (2.2), for a random sample $(y_{i1}, y_{i2}, \boldsymbol{x}_i)_{i=1}^n$, where the covariate vector $\boldsymbol{x}_i$ is the union of $\boldsymbol{x}_{i\mu_1}, \boldsymbol{x}_{i\mu_2}, \boldsymbol{x}_{i\sigma_1}, \boldsymbol{x}_{i\sigma_2}, \boldsymbol{x}_{i\nu_1}, \boldsymbol{x}_{i\nu_2}$ and $\boldsymbol{x}_{i\theta}$, the log-likelihood for the continuous outcomes copula regression model is

$$\ell(\boldsymbol{\beta}) = \sum_{i=1}^n \big[\log\{c(F_1(y_{i1}; \mu_{i1}, \sigma_{i1}, \nu_{i1}), F_2(y_{i2}; \mu_{i2}, \sigma_{i2}, \nu_{i2}); \theta_i)\}$$
$$+ \log\{f_1(y_{i1}; \mu_{i1}, \sigma_{i1}, \nu_{i1})\} + \log\{f_2(y_{i2}; \mu_{i2}, \sigma_{i2}, \nu_{i2})\}\big]$$

where $\boldsymbol{\beta} = (\boldsymbol{\beta}_{\mu_1}^\top, \boldsymbol{\beta}_{\mu_2}^\top, \boldsymbol{\beta}_{\sigma_1}^\top, \boldsymbol{\beta}_{\sigma_2}^\top, \boldsymbol{\beta}_{\nu_1}^\top, \boldsymbol{\beta}_{\nu_2}^\top, \boldsymbol{\beta}_\theta^\top)^\top$ denotes the overall regression coefficient vector.

2.4 Model fitting

The two main equations, for μ_1 and μ_2, are specified as follows

```
library(GJRM); library(GJRM.data)
data(bpc)

eq1 <- sbp ~ gender + s(bmi, by = gender) + s(mvpa) + s(sed)
eq2 <- dbp ~ gender + s(bmi, by = gender) + s(mvpa) + s(sed)
```

The remaining distributional parameters (σ_1, σ_2, ν_1, ν_2 and θ) can also be specified as functions of additive predictors using the generic formula

```
eqg <-        ~ gender + s(bmi, by = gender) + s(mvpa) + s(sed)
```

The effects of all continuous covariates are modeled flexibly, with bmi interacted with gender as this interaction was deemed the most relevant and contextually meaningful after evaluating various options.

The best marginal fits are achieved using Singh–Maddala distributions, where only μ_1 and μ_2 are specified as functions of additive predictors.

```
out1 <- gamlss(list(eq1), family = "SM", data = bpc)
out2 <- gamlss(list(eq2), family = "SM", data = bpc)
conv.check(out1); conv.check(out2)

##
## Maximum absolute gradient value: 8.637465e-08
## Observed information matrix is positive definite

##
## Maximum absolute gradient value: 6.741947e-08
## Observed information matrix is positive definite

par(mfrow = c(1,2))
res.check(out1, intervals = TRUE)
res.check(out2, intervals = TRUE)
```

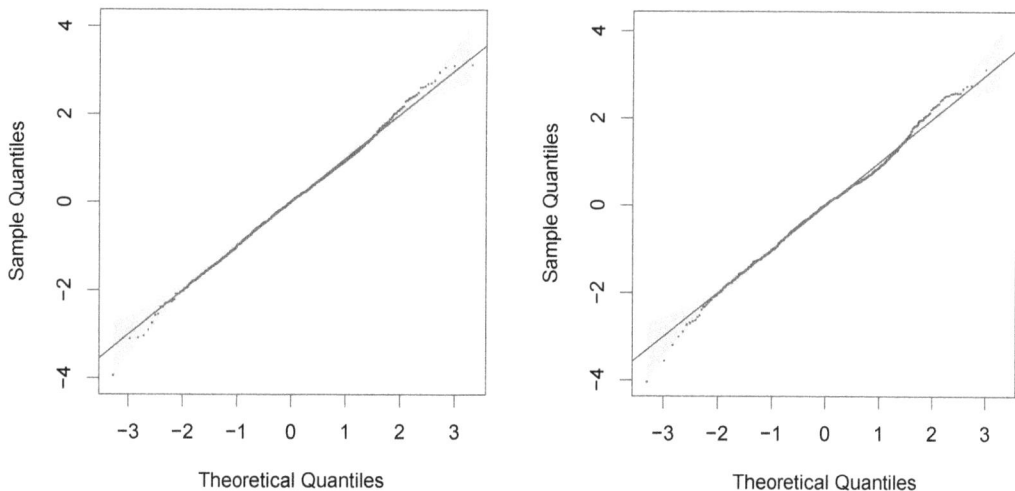

FIGURE 2.1 Normal Q–Q plots of normalized quantile residuals, derived from two additive distributional regression models with SM distribution fitted to the bpc data, using sbp (left plot) and dbp (right plot) as response variables.

Convergence checks are satisfactory and the residual plots reported in Figure 2.1 support the choice of marginal distributions. Attempts to use more complex model specifications, where σ_1, σ_2, ν_1 and ν_2 were modeled using eqg, resulted in convergence failures, suggesting that such models were too complex and not supported by the data.

Marginal means for the systolic and diastolic blood pressure levels of a child with specific features (a typical child, in this case) are shown below.

```
bpct <- data.frame(gender = 2, bmi = 18, mvpa = 55, sed = 466)

marg.mv(out1, newdata = bpct)

##
## Marginal mean with 95% interval:
##
## 105 (104,107)
marg.mv(out2, newdata = bpct)

##
## Marginal mean with 95% interval:
##
## 68.9 (67.8,70.1)
```

The difference between these two predictions is 36.1 mmHg, which falls within the typical range for normal pulse pressure (30–40 mmHg).

The next step is to fit a joint bivariate model using a Gaussian copula.

```
fl   <- list(eq1, eq2)
outN <- gjrm(fl, data = bpc, margins = c("SM", "SM"), copula = "N",
             model = "B")
outN$theta

##       theta
## 0.6533737
```

Given that the estimated correlation coefficient is positive and moderately strong, alternative copulae that align with this finding are explored. Potential candidates include C0, C180, J0, J180, G0, G180, F, T and PL. Based on convergence and information-based criteria, the Gumbel copula is selected. The more complex model specification, in which θ is modeled as a function of covariate effects using eqg, was not supported by the data.

```
outG0 <- gjrm(fl, data = bpc, margins = c("SM", "SM"), copula = "G0",
              model = "B", uni.fit = TRUE)
clarke.test(outN, outG0)

##
## Model 2 is preferred
```

The Clarke test, as well as the Vuong test (not shown here), supports the chosen copula. Comparisons with alternative copulae consistently favored the Gumbel copula.

The results from the fitted model are presented in the outputs and comments that follow.

```
summary(outG0)
```

```
##
## COPULA: Gumbel
## MARGIN 1: Singh-Maddala
## MARGIN 2: Singh-Maddala
##
## EQUATION 1
## Link function for mu1: log
## Formula: sbp ~ gender + s(bmi, by = gender) + s(mvpa) + s(sed)
##
## Parametric coefficients:
##              Estimate Std. Error z value Pr(>|z|)
## (Intercept) 4.5828617  0.0087735 522.353   <2e-16 ***
## gender2     0.0006744  0.0075573   0.089    0.929
## ---
## Signif. codes:  0 '***' 0.001 '**' 0.01 '*' 0.05 '.' 0.1 ' ' 1
##
## Approximate significance of smooth terms:
##                   edf Ref.df Chi.sq  p-value
## s(bmi):gender1 2.426  3.083 18.793 0.000347 ***
## s(bmi):gender2 3.714  4.710 18.666 0.001751 **
## s(mvpa)        1.000  1.000  0.036 0.849741
## s(sed)         1.000  1.000  0.149 0.699917
## ---
## Signif. codes:  0 '***' 0.001 '**' 0.01 '*' 0.05 '.' 0.1 ' ' 1
##
##
## EQUATION 2
## Link function for mu2: log
## Formula: dbp ~ gender + s(bmi, by = gender) + s(mvpa) + s(sed)
##
## Parametric coefficients:
##             Estimate Std. Error z value Pr(>|z|)
## (Intercept)  4.12319    0.01105 373.290   <2e-16 ***
## gender2      0.01179    0.01011   1.167    0.243
## ---
## Signif. codes:  0 '***' 0.001 '**' 0.01 '*' 0.05 '.' 0.1 ' ' 1
##
## Approximate significance of smooth terms:
##                   edf Ref.df Chi.sq p-value
## s(bmi):gender1 1.000  1.000  4.940 0.02625 *
## s(bmi):gender2 2.171  2.793 11.838 0.00576 **
## s(mvpa)        1.013  1.025  0.604 0.43794
## s(sed)         1.000  1.000  0.119 0.72979
## ---
## Signif. codes:  0 '***' 0.001 '**' 0.01 '*' 0.05 '.' 0.1 ' ' 1
##
## sigma1 = 17.1(15.2,18.4)  sigma2 = 13.2(12,14.3)
## nu1 = 0.636(0.569,0.754)  nu2 = 0.574(0.501,0.683)
## theta = 1.8(1.7,1.9)
## n = 1052  total edf = 22.3
```

The estimates indicate that `bmi` significantly affects systolic and diastolic blood pressure levels for both boys and girls, while sedentary and active times do not appear to play a major role here.

```
par(mfrow = c(2, 2))
plot(outG0, eq = 1, select = 1, scale = 0, shade = TRUE)
plot(outG0, eq = 1, select = 2, scale = 0, shade = TRUE)
plot(outG0, eq = 2, select = 1, scale = 0)
plot(outG0, eq = 2, select = 2, scale = 0)
```

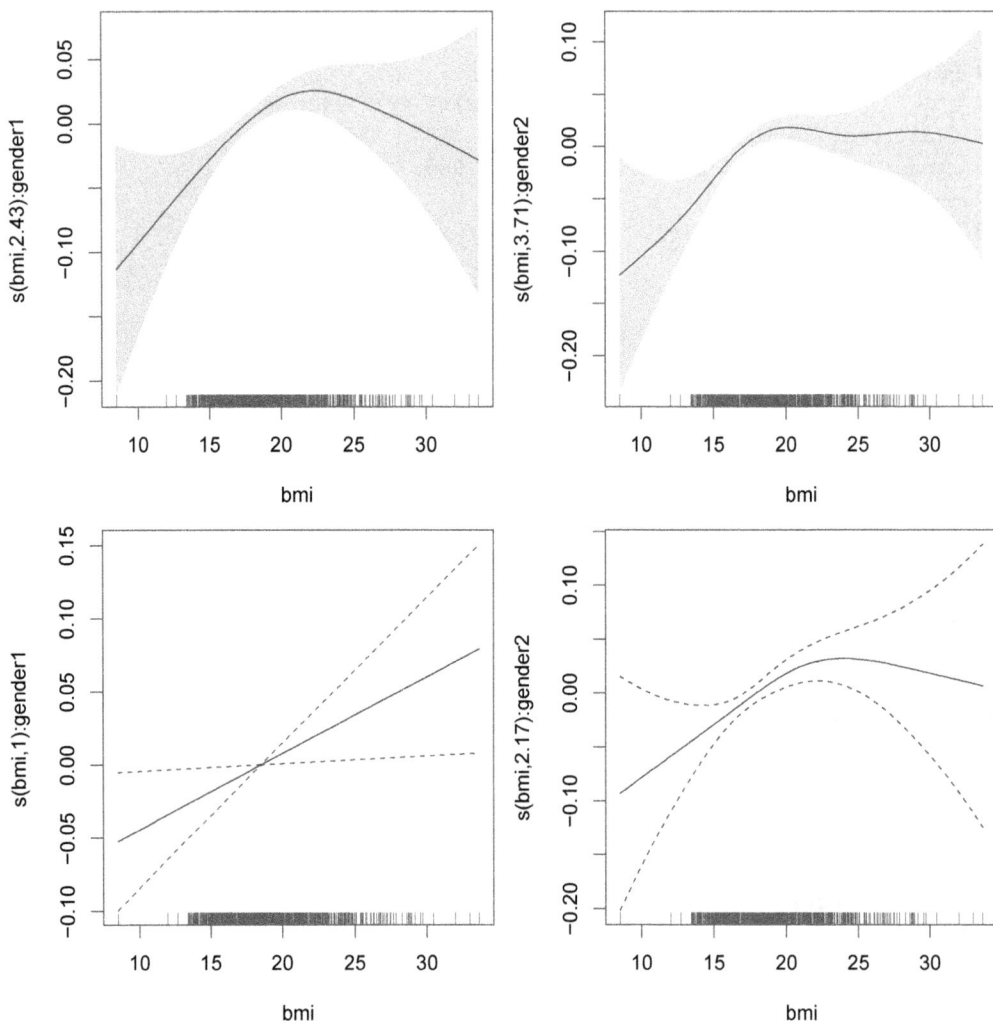

FIGURE 2.2 Estimated smooth effects (with associated 95% intervals) of `bmi` by `gender` (1 = male, 2 = female) on the scales of the additive predictors of μ_1 (top plots) and μ_2 (bottom), derived from a Gumbel copula additive distributional regression model with SM margins fitted to the `bpc` data.

The top plots in Figure 2.2 show that for boys, systolic blood pressure increases with `bmi` up to a certain point, after which it tends to decrease. In girls, systolic blood pressure rises and then levels off. However, there is greater uncertainty in the estimated effects for values of `bmi` greater than about 25. The bottom plots show that `dbp` increases with `bmi`, although this relationship weakens considerably for girls when `bmi` exceeds 24.

```
k.tau(outG0)
```

```
##       tau       2.5%      97.5%
## 0.4440977 0.4158203 0.4718411
```

The Kendall's τ reveals a significant positive residual association between systolic and diastolic blood pressures, with higher levels of one generally associated with higher levels of the other. Such a degree of dependency aligns with the common understanding that `sbp` and `dbp` typically rise together, reflecting the usual physiological relationship between these two measures.

Joint probabilities, such as $\mathbb{P}(\text{sbp} \leq 102, \text{dbp} \leq 66)$, are derived from equation (2.1).

```
copula.prob(outG0, y1 = 100, y2 = 60, newdata = bpct, intervals = TRUE)
```

```
##       p12       2.5%      97.5%
##  0.165556 0.1391452 0.1957353
```

The estimate suggests that a typical child has a 17% probability of having a systolic blood pressure of 102 mmHg or lower and a diastolic pressure of 60 mmHg or lower.

Conditional probabilities, such as $\mathbb{P}(\text{sbp} \leq 100|\text{dbp} = 60)$ and $\mathbb{P}(\text{dbp} \leq 60|\text{sbp} = 100)$, are obtained by differentiating (2.1) with respect to the marginal CDF on which the probability is conditioned.

```
copula.prob(outG0, y1 = 100, y2 = 60, cond = 2, newdata = bpct,
            intervals = TRUE)
```

```
##       p12       2.5%      97.5%
##  0.6178691 0.5590233 0.6698168
```

```
copula.prob(outG0, y1 = 100, y2 = 60, cond = 1, newdata = bpct,
            intervals = TRUE)
```

```
##       p12       2.5%      97.5%
##  0.2434435 0.2013038 0.2775699
```

The estimates indicate that for a typical child, when `dbp` is 60 mmHg, there is a 62% probability that their `sbp` will be 100 mmHg or lower. Conversely, the probability of `dbp` equal to 60 mmHg or less when `sbp` is 100 mmHg is 24%.

Conditional expectations are particularly useful in this context, and are defined as

$$\mathbb{E}(Y_2|Y_1 = y_1) = \int y_2 c(F_1(y_1; \mu_1, \sigma_1, \nu_1), F_2(y_2; \mu_2, \sigma_2, \nu_2); \theta) f_2(y_2; \mu_2, \sigma_2, \nu_2) dy_2,$$

and similarly for $\mathbb{E}(Y_1|Y_2 = y_2)$. The integration is performed over the support of y_2 (or y_1), and intervals are conveniently obtained through posterior simulation.

```
cond.mv(outG0, eq = 2, y1 = 100, newdata = bpct)
```

```
##
## Conditional mean with 95% interval:
##
## 65.3 (64.3,66.2)
```

```
cond.mv(outG0, eq = 1, y2 = 60, newdata = bpct)
```

```
##
## Conditional mean with 95% interval:
##
## 97.9 (96.4,99.3)
```

The results suggest that with sbp equal to 100 mmHg, dbp is expected to be around 65 mmHg. Conversely, with a dbp of 60 mmHg, the expected sbp is approximately 98 mmHg. Additional scenarios can be generated, making this tool particularly valuable for exploring how changes in one blood pressure impact the other.

3

Count outcomes

Applications of dependence models for count data span diverse fields such as epidemiology, medical science, insurance, marketing and sports, among others [Nikoloulopoulos and Karlis, 2010, Gurmu and Elder, 2012, Nikoloulopoulos, 2013, Shi and Valdez, 2014, Ma et al., 2017, Silva et al., 2019, Ma et al., 2020].

This chapter introduces the copula regression approach developed by van der Wurp et al. [2020] and applies it to simultaneously model visits to doctors and health professionals, while accounting for variables such as demographics, health conditions and socioeconomic status. Several post-estimation tools are employed to improve the understanding of healthcare utilization patterns.

3.1 Healthcare utilization

The empirical application uses a dataset of 10,638 observations from the 2012 Medical Expenditure Panel Survey (MEPS), collected and published by the Agency for Healthcare Research and Quality, a division of the U.S. Department of Health and Human Services. Initiated in 1996 and ongoing, the MEPS provides one of the most comprehensive individual-level databases on health insurance, healthcare usage, health conditions and socioeconomic characteristics.

In line with the analysis of Gurmu and Elder [2000], this study focuses on jointly modeling two associated outcomes: the number of consultations with a doctor (dvisit) and the number of visits to non-doctor health professionals (ndvisit). These variables exhibit overdispersion, with means and standard deviations of 2.12 and 3.6 for dvisit, and 0.94 and 2.9 for ndvisit. The available covariates are bmi, income, age, gender, ethnicity, education, region, hypertension and hyperlipidemia.

Simultaneous modeling of dvisit and ndvisit is essential given their interconnected nature: individuals who frequently visit doctors may also be more likely to consult non-doctor health professionals due to shared health conditions, for example. Furthermore, joint modeling accounts for influences, such as health-related attitudes and care preferences, that may affect both types of visits.

3.2 Model

Consider a pair of count random variables (Y_1, Y_2), where $Y_j \sim D_j(\mu_j, \sigma_j)$, for $j = 1, 2$, both modeled using the distributions in Table 1.2. The parameters are specified as $\log(\mu_j) = \eta_{\mu_j}(\mathbf{x}_{\mu_j}; \boldsymbol{\beta}_{\mu_j})$ and $\log(\sigma_j) = \eta_{\sigma_j}(\mathbf{x}_{\sigma_j}; \boldsymbol{\beta}_{\sigma_j})$.

DOI: 10.1201/9781003593195-3

The joint CDF of Y_1 and Y_2 is expressed as

$$\mathbb{P}(Y_1 \leq y_1, \ Y_2 \leq y_2) = C(F_1(y_1; \mu_1, \sigma_1), \ F_2(y_2; \mu_2, \sigma_2); \theta),$$

where $F_j(y_j; \mu_j, \sigma_j)$ is the marginal CDF of Y_j and $C(\cdot, \cdot; \theta)$ is a copula function with dependence parameter $g_\theta(\theta) = \eta_\theta(\mathbf{x}_\theta; \boldsymbol{\beta}_\theta)$.

The joint PMF is

$$\begin{aligned}
f_{12}(y_1, y_2; \mu_1, \mu_2, \sigma_1, \sigma_2, \theta) = {} & C(F_1(y_1; \mu_1, \sigma_1), F_2(y_2; \mu_2, \sigma_2); \theta) \\
& - C(F_1(y_1 - 1; \mu_1, \sigma_1), F_2(y_2; \mu_2, \sigma_2)) \\
& - C(F_1(y_1; \mu_1, \sigma_1), F_2(y_2 - 1; \mu_2, \sigma_2); \theta) \\
& + C(F_1(y_1 - 1; \mu_1, \sigma_1), F_2(y_2 - 1; \mu_2, \sigma_2); \theta)
\end{aligned} \tag{3.1}$$

When evaluating (3.1), $F_j(y_j - 1; \mu_j, \sigma_j)$ is replaced with $F_j(y_j; \mu_j, \sigma_j) - f_j(y_j; \mu_j, \sigma_j)$, where $f_j(y_j; \mu_j, \sigma_j)$ is the jth marginal PMF. This adjustment is particularly relevant for the case $y_j = 0$, where $F_j(-1; \mu_j, \sigma_j)$ has to be set to 0.

3.3   Log-likelihood

Using equation (3.1), for a random sample $\{(y_{i1}, y_{i2}, \boldsymbol{x}_i)\}_{i=1}^n$, where the covariate vector $\boldsymbol{x}_i$ is the union of $\boldsymbol{x}_{i\mu_1}$, $\boldsymbol{x}_{i\mu_2}$, $\boldsymbol{x}_{i\sigma_1}$, $\boldsymbol{x}_{i\sigma_2}$ and $\boldsymbol{x}_{i\theta}$, the log-likelihood of the count outcomes copula regression model is

$$\ell(\boldsymbol{\beta}) = \sum_{i=1}^n \log f_{12}(y_{i1}, y_{i2}; \mu_{i1}, \mu_{i2}, \sigma_{i1}, \sigma_{i2}, \theta_i),$$

where $\boldsymbol{\beta} = (\boldsymbol{\beta}_{\mu_1}^\top, \boldsymbol{\beta}_{\mu_2}^\top, \boldsymbol{\beta}_{\sigma_1}^\top, \boldsymbol{\beta}_{\sigma_2}^\top, \boldsymbol{\beta}_\theta^\top)^\top$ is the overall regression coefficient vector.

3.4   Model fitting

A number of model specifications were considered, using various copulae (starting with the Gaussian), count marginal distributions and additive predictors for all the distributional parameters. Based on convergence and residual checks, information-based criteria as well as considerations of parsimony and the estimated *edf* values for the smooths of bmi, income, age and education, the preferred model is

```
library(GJRM); library(GJRM.data)
data(meps)
eq1 <- dvisit  ~ bmi + s(income) + age + education + ethnicity +
                 region + gender + hypertension + hyperlipidemia
eq2 <- ndvisit ~ bmi + income + age + education + ethnicity +
                 region + gender + hypertension + hyperlipidemia

out <- gjrm(list(eq1, eq2), margins = c("NBII", "PIG"), copula = "N",
            data = meps, model = "B", uni.fit = TRUE)
```

```
conv.check(out)
```

```
##
## Maximum absolute gradient value: 0.002884703
## Observed information matrix is positive definite
res.check(out, intervals = TRUE)
```

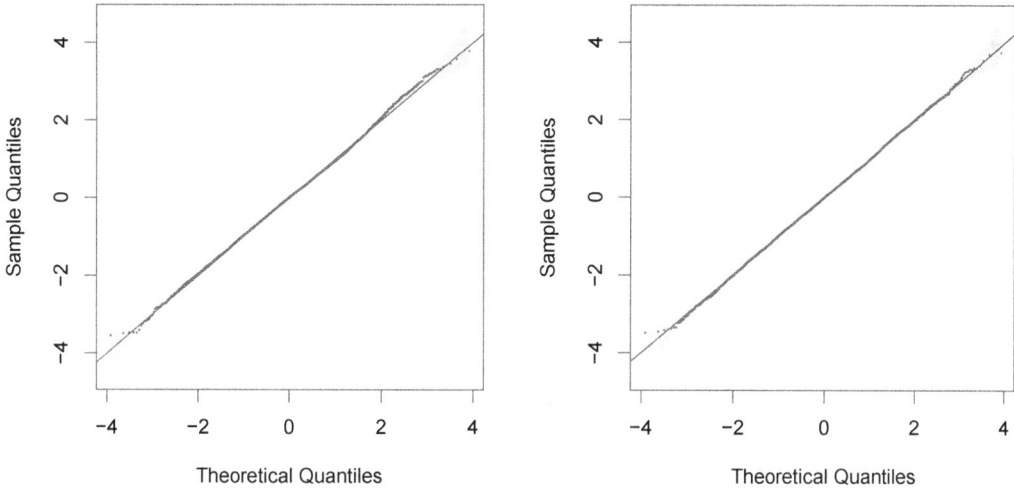

FIGURE 3.1 Normal Q–Q plots of randomized normalized quantile residuals, derived from a Gaussian copula additive distributional regression model with NBII and PIG margins fitted to the meps data.

Convergence checks are adequate, and the residual plots reported in Figure 3.1 support the choice of marginal distributions. This is not surprising given that the two count outcomes are overdispersed (as pointed out in Section 3.1), making more classical options, such as the Poisson, unsuitable for these data.

Marginal means for dvisit and ndvisit of an individual with specific attributes (a typical subject, in this case) are given below.

```
nd <- data.frame(bmi = 27, income = 47000, age = 40, gender = 0,
                 ethnicity = 1, region = 3, education = 12,
                 hypertension = 0, hyperlipidemia = 0)
```

```
marg.mv(out, eq = 1, newdata = nd)
```

```
##
## Marginal mean with 95% interval:
##
## 1.74 (1.65,1.85)
marg.mv(out, eq = 2, newdata = nd)
```

```
##
## Marginal mean with 95% interval:
##
## 0.533 (0.478,0.581)
```

On average, this individual is expected to visit a doctor 1.7 times and consult non-doctor health professionals 0.5 times. This difference likely reflects the broader trend of seeking medical care from doctors more frequently than from other health professionals, possibly due to perceived expertise and the nature of primary care needs.

The results from the fitted model are summarized in the following outputs and comments.

```
summary(out)
```

```
##
## COPULA: Gaussian
## MARGIN 1: Negative Binomial - Type II
## MARGIN 2: Poisson Inverse Gaussian
##
## EQUATION 1
## Link function for mu1: log
## Formula: dvisit ~ bmi + s(income) + age + education + ethnicity + region +
##     gender + hypertension + hyperlipidemia
##
## Parametric coefficients:
##                 Estimate Std. Error z value Pr(>|z|)
## (Intercept)    -0.844761   0.098984  -8.534  < 2e-16 ***
## bmi             0.013115   0.001880   6.977 3.02e-12 ***
## age             0.014235   0.001060  13.431  < 2e-16 ***
## education       0.053407   0.004736  11.277  < 2e-16 ***
## ethnicity2     -0.153882   0.031923  -4.820 1.43e-06 ***
## ethnicity3     -0.008676   0.128480  -0.068  0.94616
## ethnicity4     -0.196370   0.046899  -4.187 2.83e-05 ***
## region2         0.049234   0.039459   1.248  0.21212
## region3        -0.103972   0.035900  -2.896  0.00378 **
## region4        -0.122555   0.038960  -3.146  0.00166 **
## gender         -0.574581   0.025331 -22.683  < 2e-16 ***
## hypertension    0.370181   0.030061  12.315  < 2e-16 ***
## hyperlipidemia  0.446272   0.029639  15.057  < 2e-16 ***
## ---
## Signif. codes:  0 '***' 0.001 '**' 0.01 '*' 0.05 '.' 0.1 ' ' 1
##
## Approximate significance of smooth terms:
##            edf Ref.df Chi.sq p-value
## s(income) 4.916  6.024  35.46  <2e-16 ***
## ---
## Signif. codes:  0 '***' 0.001 '**' 0.01 '*' 0.05 '.' 0.1 ' ' 1
##
##
## EQUATION 2
## Link function for mu2: log
## Formula: ndvisit ~ bmi + income + age + education + ethnicity + region +
##     gender + hypertension + hyperlipidemia
##
## Parametric coefficients:
##                 Estimate Std. Error z value Pr(>|z|)
## (Intercept)    -3.707e+00  2.257e-01 -16.424  < 2e-16 ***
```

```
## bmi             1.560e-02  4.602e-03   3.390 0.000699 ***
## income          2.187e-06  5.848e-07   3.740 0.000184 ***
## age             1.916e-02  2.470e-03   7.758 8.60e-15 ***
## education       1.785e-01  1.154e-02  15.464  < 2e-16 ***
## ethnicity2      -5.603e-01  8.099e-02  -6.918 4.57e-12 ***
## ethnicity3      -3.836e-02  3.358e-01  -0.114 0.909066
## ethnicity4      -4.122e-01  1.042e-01  -3.956 7.61e-05 ***
## region2          5.241e-01  9.545e-02   5.491 3.99e-08 ***
## region3         -3.539e-01  8.902e-02  -3.975 7.03e-05 ***
## region4          3.720e-01  9.223e-02   4.034 5.49e-05 ***
## gender          -8.847e-01  6.017e-02 -14.705  < 2e-16 ***
## hypertension     3.483e-01  7.513e-02   4.636 3.55e-06 ***
## hyperlipidemia   6.286e-01  7.385e-02   8.512  < 2e-16 ***
## ---
## Signif. codes:  0 '***' 0.001 '**' 0.01 '*' 0.05 '.' 0.1 ' ' 1
##
## sigma1 = 3.84(3.69,4.05)  sigma2 = 12.9(11.5,14.4)
## theta = 0.426(0.406,0.447)
## n = 10638   total edf = 34.9
```

All the covariates play a significant role in predicting both doctor and non-doctor health professional visits, highlighting the multifaceted nature of healthcare utilization. Most effects align with expected patterns in this research field. For example, older `age` and higher `bmi` are associated with increased healthcare visits. Specifically, an increase of one unit in `bmi` leads to approximately a 1.3% increase in the average number of doctor consultations and a 1.6% increase in non-doctor visits, holding the other variables constant. Significant differences by `gender`, `ethnicity` and `region` further underscore the influence of demographic characteristics on healthcare utilization, which may inform tailored health services and interventions. For instance, males are expected to make about 44% fewer doctor consultations and 59% fewer non-doctor visits compared to females. Similar interpretations apply to the other covariate effects.

```
plot(out, eq = 1, rug = TRUE, jit = TRUE)
```

Figure 3.2 illustrates that as `income` increases, `dvisit` decreases for `income` levels up to approximately $50,000. Beyond this point, for `income` values between $50,000 and $200,000, the number of doctor visits begins to increase. For very high `income` levels, the relationship between `income` and `dvisit` is less reliably estimated due to the sparsity of the data. The findings suggest that lower-income individuals might face barriers that reduce their frequency of doctor visits, while middle and higher-income individuals might have better access and more frequent engagement with healthcare services. This highlights the importance of optimizing resource allocation as well as developing tailored healthcare policies and interventions that address the unique needs of each income group and ensure equitable access to healthcare.

The estimated correlation coefficient is positive and statistically significant, which suggests that after controlling for covariates, the two responses share some individual-level heterogeneity (e.g., personal preferences and lifestyle choices) that drives both doctor and non-doctor visits.

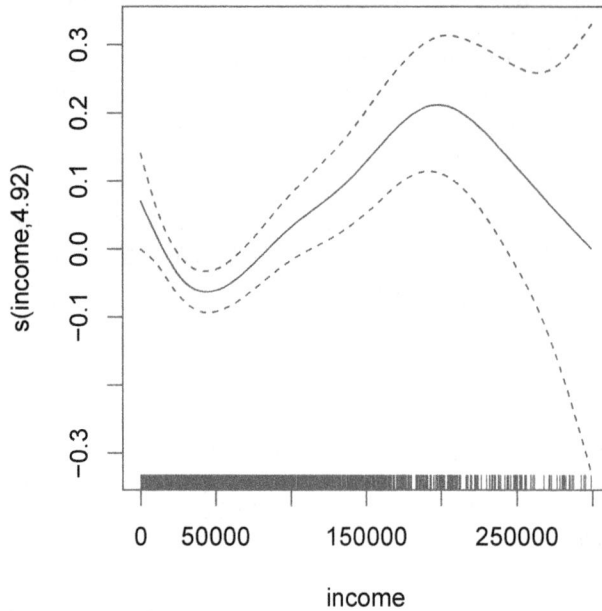

FIGURE 3.2 Estimated smooth effect (with associated 95% intervals) of `income` on the scale of the additive predictor of μ_1, derived from a Gaussian copula additive distributional regression model with `NBII` and `PIG` margins fitted to the `meps` data.

For a typical individual, joint probability estimates, such as $\mathbb{P}(\text{dvisit} = 0, \text{ndvisit} = 0)$, are computed using (3.1).

```
copula.prob(out, y1 = 0, y2 = 0, newdata = nd, intervals = TRUE)
```

```
##         p12        2.5%       97.5%
##   0.4402936 0.4214075 0.4606869
```

```
copula.prob(out, y1 = 0, y2 = 0, newdata = nd, joint = FALSE,
            intervals = TRUE)
```

```
##         p12        2.5%       97.5%
##   0.3951881 0.3775654 0.4098861
```

The estimates from the copula model and from the model assuming independence of the margins differ significantly, with the former providing a more realistic estimate, given the heterogeneity captured by the correlation coefficient.

Conditional probabilities, such as $\mathbb{P}(\text{dvisit} = 2|\text{ndvisit} = 1)$ and $\mathbb{P}(\text{ndvisit} = 2|\text{dvisit} = 3)$, are given by the ratio between (3.1) and the marginal PMF on which the probability is conditioned.

```
copula.prob(out, y1 = 2, y2 = 1, cond = 2, newdata = nd, intervals = TRUE)
```

```
##         p12      2.5%       97.5%
##   0.1307696 0.12794 0.1349833
```

```
copula.prob(out, y1 = 2, y2 = 1, cond = 2, newdata = nd, joint = FALSE,
            intervals = TRUE)
```

```
##          p12        2.5%      97.5%
##   0.1009481 0.09698881 0.1049757
```

```
copula.prob(out, y1 = 3, y2 = 2, cond = 1, newdata = nd, intervals = TRUE)
```

```
##          p12       2.5%      97.5%
##   0.05171865 0.0472458 0.05541095
```

```
copula.prob(out, y1 = 3, y2 = 2, cond = 1, newdata = nd, joint = FALSE,
            intervals = TRUE)
```

```
##          p12        2.5%      97.5%
##   0.03371129 0.03176489 0.03716757
```

These results suggest that non-doctor visits modestly affect the likelihood of doctor visits, and vice versa. Specifically, the probability of having two doctor visits given one non-doctor visit is 13% when taking into account dependence, compared to 10% under the assumption of independence. Conversely, the probability of having two non-doctor visits given three doctor visits is 5% when dependence is accounted for and 3% when it is not.

Conditional expectations offer further insights into the relationship between the two responses. They are defined as

$$\mathbb{E}(Y_2|Y_1 = y_1) = \frac{1}{f_1(y_1;\mu_1,\sigma_1)} \sum_{y_2=1}^{\infty} y_2 f_{12}(y_1, y_2; \mu_1, \mu_2, \sigma_1, \sigma_2, \theta), \qquad (3.2)$$

and similarly for $\mathbb{E}(Y_1|Y_2 = y_2)$. Intervals are conveniently obtained through posterior simulation. Expression (3.2) is approximated by summing up to a specified limit for y_2 (or y_1) beyond which additional outcomes have negligible impact on the overall sum. For a typical subject and illustrative values of the conditioning variables, the conditional means are provided in the following outputs.

```
cond.mv(out, eq = 1, y2 = 2, newdata = nd)
```

```
##
## Conditional mean with 95% interval:
##
## 3.45 (3.20,3.66)
```

```
cond.mv(out, eq = 2, y1 = 5, newdata = nd)
```

```
##
## Conditional mean with 95% interval:
##
## 1.112 (0.981,1.249)
```

They indicate that a typical individual with two non-doctor visits can expect about 3.5 doctor visits and that an individual with five doctor visits is expected to have about one non-doctor visit.

4

Survival outcomes

In research areas such as medicine, biology and insurance, bivariate survival outcomes are frequently analyzed. For instance, in HIV/AIDS studies, researchers often explore the relationship between the time from antiretroviral therapy (ART) initiation to viral failure and the time from ART initiation to regimen change [Eden et al., 2022]. In oncology, investigations may focus on the time from birth to cancer onset and the time from cancer onset to death [Zhu and Wang, 2012]. In actuarial science, bivariate survival analysis may be employed to examine the dependence of death times for coupled lives using data from life annuity portfolios [Carriere, 2000].

The copula additive distributional regression framework accommodates bivariate survival outcomes while addressing the unique challenges posed by various types of censoring, including right, left and interval censoring [Marra and Radice, 2020]. A case study on age-related macular degeneration (AMD) illustrates this method, as the progression times in both eyes are dependent. The analysis demonstrates how the copula survival regression model effectively captures the dependence between the progression times while handling different censoring mechanisms and flexibly incorporating covariate effects. Furthermore, the model enables the prediction of progression-free survival for specific patient profiles.

4.1 Age-related eye disease

The empirical application uses data from the Age-Related Eye Disease Study (AREDS), a multicenter randomized clinical trial sponsored by the National Eye Institute, investigating the development and progression of AMD [AREDS Group, 1999]. The analysis aims to quantify the effects of clinical variables on the risk of AMD progression in the left and right eyes, and to predict the progression profiles of patients with different characteristics. The dataset includes information from 628 subjects on the times (in years) to late-stage AMD in both eyes, which are either interval or right-censored, along with three covariates: baseline severity score, age and a genetic variant.

Jointly modeling the AMD progression times within a regression framework is essential because both eyes share the same risk factors, such as genetic predisposition, age, environmental influences and personal habits. Furthermore, joint modeling improves the prediction of progression profiles, helping to identify individuals at higher risk of rapid deterioration, ultimately supporting better clinical decision-making.

DOI: 10.1201/9781003593195-4

4.2   Model

Consider a pair of survival times (Y_1, Y_2) and their corresponding survival functions

$$S_j\,(y_j) = g_{S_j}^{-1}\left\{\eta_{S_j}(\boldsymbol{x}_{S_j};\boldsymbol{\beta}_{S_j})\right\},\ j = 1, 2,$$

where $g_{S_j}(\cdot)$ is a link function and $\eta_{S_j}(\boldsymbol{x}_{S_j};\boldsymbol{\beta}_{S_j})$ is an additive predictor that depends on $\boldsymbol{x}_{S_j} = \left(y_j, \boldsymbol{x}_{\mu_j}^\top\right)^\top$ and $\boldsymbol{\beta}_{S_j}$ (see Section 1.1.1).

The joint survival function $S(y_1, y_2) = \mathbb{P}(Y_1 > y_1, Y_2 > y_2)$ can be represented as

$$C\left(S_1(y_1), S_2(y_2); \theta\right),\tag{4.1}$$

where $C(\cdot, \cdot; \theta)$ is a copula function with $g_\theta(\theta) = \eta_\theta(\boldsymbol{x}_\theta; \boldsymbol{\beta}_\theta)$.

In the presence of censoring, Y_j is only known to lie within the interval (L_{cj}, R_{cj}), where L_{cj} and R_{cj} represent the left and right censoring times, respectively. If $L_{cj} = 0$, the observation for the jth margin is classified as left-censored. When $R_{cj} = \infty$, the observation is considered right-censored. If L_{cj} and R_{cj} take finite, distinct, non-zero values, the observation is interval-censored. Uncensored observations occur when $L_{cj} = R_{cj}$. Consequently, there are 16 possible censoring combinations to account for, which can be distinguished using the indicator functions δ_{I_j} and δ_{U_j}. Here, $\delta_{I_j} = 1$ if the observation is interval-, right- or left-censored and 0 otherwise, while $\delta_{U_j} = 1$ if the observation is uncensored and 0 otherwise.

4.3   Log-likelihood

For a random sample $(l_{ci1}, l_{ci2}, r_{ci1}, r_{ci2}, \boldsymbol{x}_i)_{i=1}^n$, where the covariate vector $\boldsymbol{x}_i$ is the union of $\boldsymbol{x}_{iS_1}$, $\boldsymbol{x}_{iS_2}$ and $\boldsymbol{x}_{i\theta}$, the log-likelihood function of the survival copula regression model with mixed censoring mechanisms is

$$\begin{aligned}
\ell(\boldsymbol{\beta}) = {}& \delta_{U_{i1}}\delta_{U_{i2}}\sum_{i=1}^n \log\left[\frac{\partial^2}{\partial y_{i1}\partial y_{i2}}C\left\{S_1(y_{i1}), S_2(y_{i2});\theta_i\right\}\right]\\
& + \delta_{I_{i1}}\delta_{I_{i2}}\sum_{i=1}^n \log\Big[C\{S_1(l_{ci1}), S_2(l_{ci2});\theta_i\} - C\{S_1(l_{ci1}), S_2(r_{ci2});\theta_i\}\\
& \qquad - C\{S_1(r_{ci1}), S_2(l_{ci2});\theta_i\} + C\{S_1(r_{ci1}), S_2(r_{ci2});\theta_i\}\Big]\\
& + \delta_{U_{i1}}\delta_{I_{i2}}\sum_{i=1}^n \log\left[\frac{\partial}{\partial y_{i1}}\Big(C\{S_1(y_{i1}), S_2(r_{ci2});\theta_i\} - C\{S_1(y_{i1}), S_2(l_{ci2});\theta_i\}\Big)\right]\\
& + \delta_{I_{i1}}\delta_{U_{i2}}\sum_{i=1}^n \log\left[\frac{\partial}{\partial y_{i2}}\Big(C\{S_1(r_{ci1}), S_2(y_{i2});\theta_i\} - C\{S_1(l_{ci1}), S_2(y_{i2});\theta_i\}\Big)\right]
\end{aligned},$$

where $\boldsymbol{\beta} = (\boldsymbol{\beta}_{S_1}^\top, \boldsymbol{\beta}_{S_2}^\top, \boldsymbol{\beta}_\theta^\top)^\top$ is the overall regression coefficient vector. If an observation is uncensored, then $l_{cij} = r_{cij} = y_{ij}$.

4.4   Model fitting

The equations for the survival outcomes are specified as

```
library(GJRM); library(GJRM.data)
data(areds)

eq1 <- t11 ~ s(log(t11), bs = "mpi") + s(age) + SevScore1 + rs2284665
eq2 <- t21 ~ s(log(t21), bs = "mpi") + s(age) + SevScore2 + rs2284665
```

where the negative of the baseline survival function and the impacts of `age` are modeled flexibly. Note that smoothing of `t11` and `t21` is implemented on log-transformed times. Although not required, this helps obtain smoother estimated survival functions.

The dependence parameter is also specified as a function of an additive predictor, using the following equation

```
eq3 <-      ~ s(age) + rs2284665
```

More complex regression structures, including interaction effects such as `ti(log(t11), age)` and `s(log(t11), by = rs2284665)`, either led to converge failures or were not supported by information-based criteria, suggesting that these specifications were too complex for the data at hand.

For a given copula structure (in this case, Gaussian), the functions $g_{S_j}(\cdot)$ were selected by comparing the nine models resulting from all possible combinations of links available. For both margins, `-logit` emerged as the most preferred choice.

The next step is to fit a joint survival regression model with `-logit` margins and a Gaussian copula.

```
fl  <- list(eq1, eq2, eq3)
outN <- gjrm(fl, data = areds, margins = c("-logit", "-logit"),
             copula = "N", cens1 = cens1, cens2 = cens2,
             ub.t1 = "t12", ub.t2 = "t22", model = "B")
conv.check(outN)

##
## Maximum absolute gradient value: 5.739132e-09
## Observed information matrix is positive definite
```

Convergence checks are satisfactory, while the summary output for the θ equation (shown below) suggests that the covariates have a weak influence on the dependence parameter. Therefore, the model can be simplified.

```
summary(outN)

...
## EQUATION 3
## Link function for theta: atanh
## Formula: ~s(age) + rs2284665
##
## Parametric coefficients:
##               Estimate Std. Error z value Pr(>|z|)
```

```
## (Intercept)    0.45902    0.08301   5.530 3.21e-08 ***
## rs22846651     0.17395    0.10767   1.616    0.106
## rs22846652     0.15126    0.14560   1.039    0.299
## ---
## Signif. codes:  0 '***' 0.001 '**' 0.01 '*' 0.05 '.' 0.1 ' ' 1
##
## Approximate significance of smooth terms:
##          edf Ref.df Chi.sq p-value
## s(age) 1.611  2.016  1.166   0.556
##
## theta = 0.507(0.353,0.639)
...
```

Since the correlation coefficient is positive and reasonably strong, it is sensible to evaluate only alternative copulae that are consistent with this finding (e.g., C0, C180, J0, J180, G0, G180, F, T, PL). Based on convergence and information-based criteria, the Plackett is selected.

```
fl   <- list(eq1, eq2)
outPL <- gjrm(fl, data = areds, margins = c("-logit", "-logit"),
              copula = "PL", cens1 = cens1, cens2 = cens2,
              ub.t1 = "t12", ub.t2 = "t22", model = "B")
vuong.test(outN, outPL)
```

```
##
## Model 2 is preferred
```

The Vuong test, as well as the Clarke test (not shown here), supports the chosen copula. Comparisons with alternative copulae consistently favored the Plackett.

The findings are explored in the outputs and discussion that follow.

```
k.tau(outPL)
```

```
##        tau      2.5%     97.5%
## 0.3568872 0.2988751 0.4150041
```

A Kendall's τ of 0.36 indicates a moderate positive association between the progression to late-stage AMD in both eyes. This dependence suggests that after accounting for covariates, influences, such as genetic predispositions, inflammatory responses and vascular variables, also play a role in explaining the progression times. Clinically, this highlights the importance of closely monitoring both eyes simultaneously, as the health of one eye can provide valuable insights into the risk of disease progression in the other.

```
summary(outPL)
```

```
##
## COPULA: Plackett
## MARGIN 1: Survival with -logit link
## MARGIN 2: Survival with -logit link
##
## EQUATION 1
## Formula: t11 ~ s(log(t11), bs = "mpi") + s(age) + SevScore1 + rs2284665
##
## Parametric coefficients:
##               Estimate Std. Error z value Pr(>|z|)
```

```
## (Intercept)   -2.7550   0.4748  -5.802 6.53e-09 ***
## SevScore15      0.6587   0.2406   2.737  0.00619 **
## SevScore16      0.9860   0.2226   4.429 9.48e-06 ***
## SevScore17      1.9046   0.2301   8.278  < 2e-16 ***
## SevScore18      2.8246   0.3166   8.922  < 2e-16 ***
## rs22846651      0.3249   0.1665   1.951  0.05101 .
## rs22846652      0.5999   0.2327   2.578  0.00993 **
## ---
## Signif. codes:  0 '***' 0.001 '**' 0.01 '*' 0.05 '.' 0.1 ' ' 1
##
## Approximate significance of smooth terms:
##                 edf Ref.df Chi.sq p-value
## s(log(t11)) 2.525  3.136 4270.9 < 2e-16 ***
## s(age)      1.602  2.004   12.6 0.00184 **
## ---
## Signif. codes:  0 '***' 0.001 '**' 0.01 '*' 0.05 '.' 0.1 ' ' 1
##
##
## EQUATION 2
## Formula: t21 ~ s(log(t21), bs = "mpi") + s(age) + SevScore2 + rs2284665
##
## Parametric coefficients:
##               Estimate Std. Error z value Pr(>|z|)
## (Intercept)   -3.3902     0.7515  -4.511 6.45e-06 ***
## SevScore25      0.8067     0.2547   3.168 0.001537 **
## SevScore26      1.1863     0.2385   4.974 6.55e-07 ***
## SevScore27      2.4076     0.2520   9.554  < 2e-16 ***
## SevScore28      3.2745     0.3299   9.926  < 2e-16 ***
## rs22846651      0.4573     0.1683   2.717 0.006591 **
## rs22846652      0.7826     0.2253   3.474 0.000513 ***
## ---
## Signif. codes:  0 '***' 0.001 '**' 0.01 '*' 0.05 '.' 0.1 ' ' 1
##
## Approximate significance of smooth terms:
##                 edf Ref.df  Chi.sq p-value
## s(log(t21)) 2.14  2.526 4947.569  <2e-16 ***
## s(age)      1.00  1.000    6.187  0.0129 *
## ---
## Signif. codes:  0 '***' 0.001 '**' 0.01 '*' 0.05 '.' 0.1 ' ' 1
##
## theta = 5.27(4.06,6.91)
## n = 628  total edf = 22.3
```

Considering the left eye and the impact of the severity score variable, the odds ratios for progression to late-stage AMD within the interval $(0, t]$ are estimated as follows: $\exp(0.6587) \approx 1.9$ for SevScore1 = 5, 2.7 for SevScore1 = 6, 6.7 for SevScore1 = 7 and 16.9 for SevScore1 = 8, compared with SevScore1 = 4. This shows a clear, positive relationship between severity score and the probability of progressing to late-stage AMD, with the risk of progression rising significantly as the severity score increases. The odds ratios for genetic variants 1 and 2 are 1.4 and 1.8, respectively, compared to genetic variant 0. This suggests that both variants are associated with higher risks of AMD progression compared to variant 0, with variant 2 having a stronger effect. Similar patterns are observed for the right eye.

```
par(mfrow = c(1, 2))
plot(outPL, eq = 1, scale = 0, select = 2, rug = TRUE)
plot(outPL, eq = 2, scale = 0, select = 2, rug = TRUE)
```

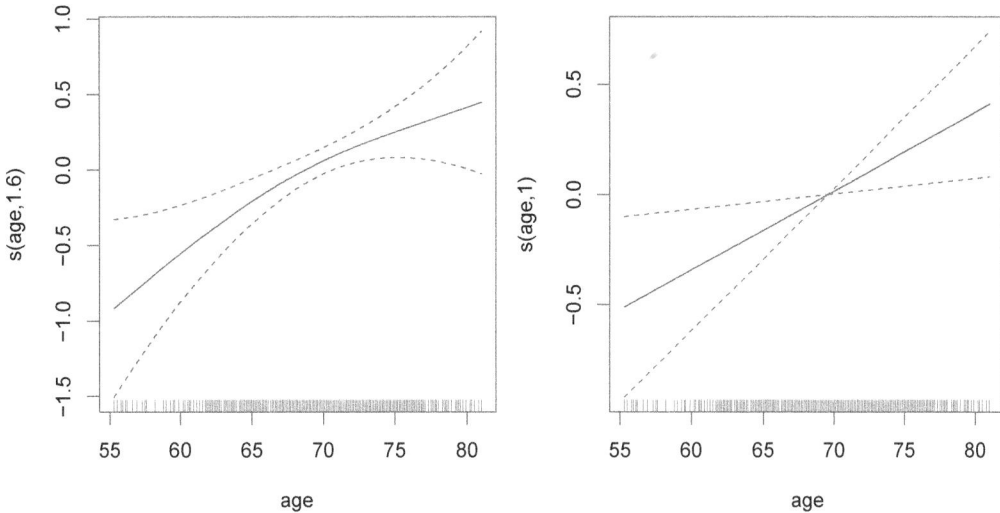

FIGURE 4.1 Estimated smooth effects (with associated 95% intervals) of `age` on the scales of the additive predictors of the survival functions for the left and right eyes, derived from a Plackett survival additive distributional regression model with `-logit` margins fitted to the `areds` data.

Figure 4.1 suggests that as `age` increases, the hazard of late-stage AMD rises for both the left and right eyes. However, because these effects are presented on the scales of the additive predictors and are therefore not directly interpretable, Figure 4.2 provides an alternative plot, for the left eye of a typical patient profile. Another example is displayed in Figure 4.3, for the right eye, whose results align with the estimated odds ratios discussed earlier.

Estimated survival, hazard and cumulative hazard functions for both eyes, for a typical individual (`age` = 69, `SevScore1` = 7, `SevScore2` = 6, `rs2284665` = 1), can be displayed using various options, as shown in Figure 4.4.

```
par(mfrow = c(2, 3), cex.lab = 1.5)
nd <- data.frame(age = 69, SevScore1 = 7, SevScore2 = 6, rs2284665 = 1)

haz.surv(outPL, eq = 1, newdata = nd,  bars = TRUE, type = "surv")
haz.surv(outPL, eq = 1, newdata = nd, shade = TRUE, type = "haz",
         baseline = TRUE, ylab = "Baseline hazard", t.range = c(2, 10))
haz.surv(outPL, eq = 1, newdata = nd, shade = TRUE, type = "cum.haz")
haz.surv(outPL, eq = 2, newdata = nd, type = "surv")
haz.surv(outPL, eq = 2, newdata = nd,  bars = TRUE, type = "haz",
         t.vec = c(0.5, 3, 6, 8))
haz.surv(outPL, eq = 2, newdata = nd, type = "cum.haz",
         baseline = TRUE, ylab = "Baseline cumulative hazard")
```

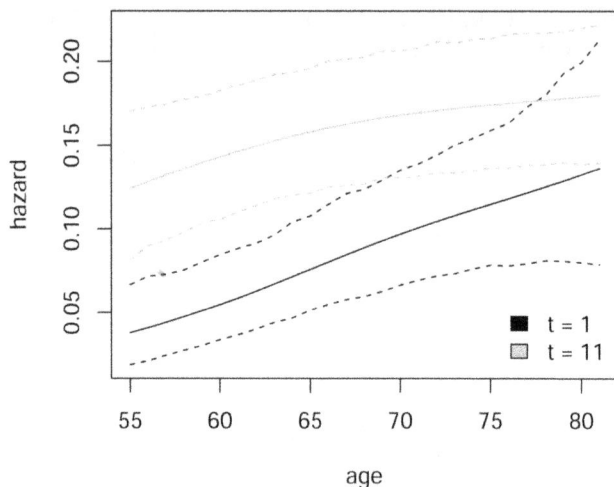

FIGURE 4.2 Impact of `age` on the hazard of late-stage AMD (with associated 95% intervals) at two time points, for the left eye, calculated using typical values of `SevScore1` and `rs2284665`.

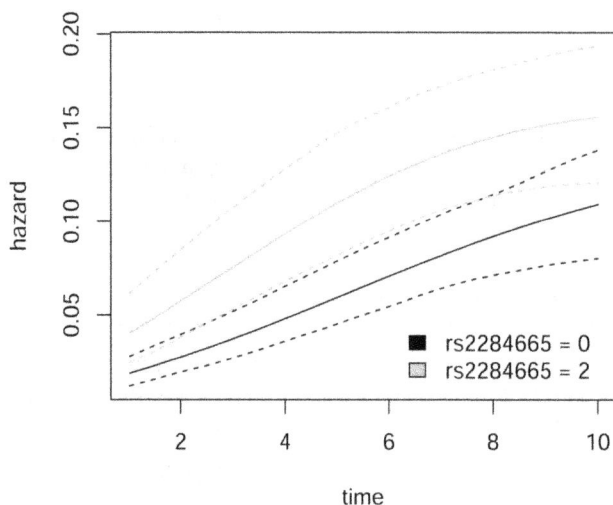

FIGURE 4.3 Hazard functions for late-stage AMD (with associated 95% intervals) by `rs2284665` (0 and 2) for the right eye, calculated using typical values of `SevScore2` and `age`.

Joint survival probabilities at specific time points, such as $\mathbb{P}(\texttt{t11} > 4, \texttt{t21} > 4)$, are calculated using (4.1).

```
nd <- data.frame(t11 = 4, t21 = 4, age = 69, SevScore1 = 7, SevScore2 = 6,
                 rs2284665 = 1)
copula.prob(outPL, newdata = nd, intervals = TRUE)

##         p12       2.5%      97.5%
##   0.5957098 0.4841883 0.6500312
```

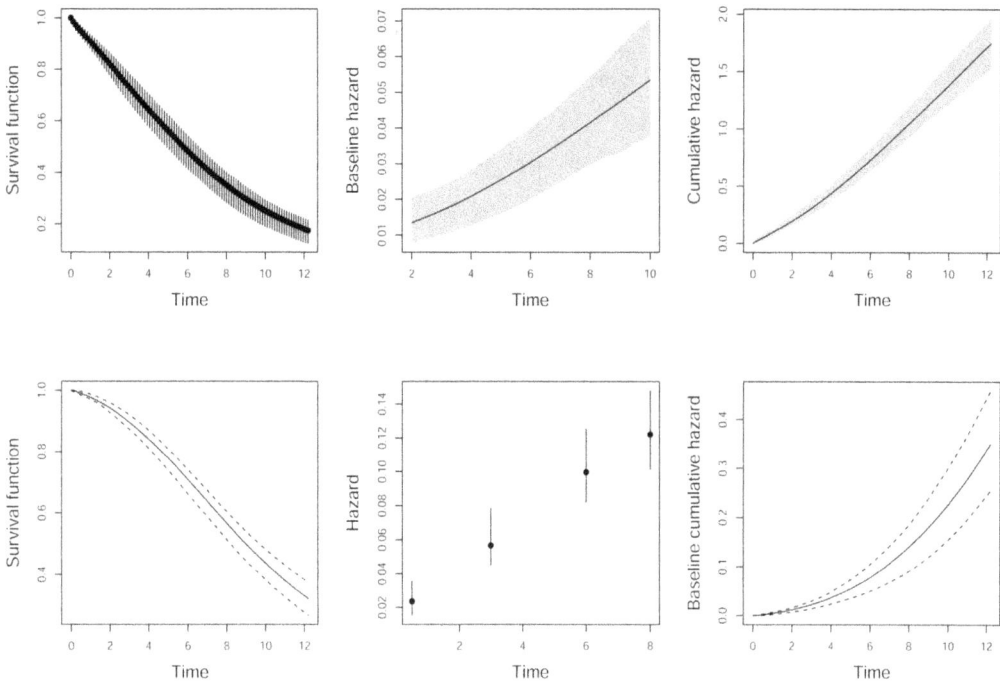

FIGURE 4.4 Estimated survival, (baseline) hazard and (baseline) cumulative hazard functions (with associated 95% intervals) for a typical individual, for the left (top plots) and right (bottom plots) eyes, derived from a Plackett survival additive distributional regression model with `-logit` margins fitted to the `areds` data.

```
nd$age   <- 40
copula.prob(outPL, newdata = nd, intervals = TRUE)

##          p12       2.5%      97.5%
##    0.8896322 0.6353807 0.9424504
```

The estimates indicate that the progression-free probability for the left and right eyes at time 4 is about 60% and that this probability increases to 89% when `age = 40`.

For a typical subject, a comprehensive view of the joint probabilities is provided in Figure 4.5. The plots show that the estimates derived from the dependence model are generally higher compared to those obtained under the assumption of independence of the margins, although both graphs exhibit similar patterns. The higher probabilities from the copula model highlight the need to account for dependence when assessing the risk of AMD progression.

Conditional survival probabilities, such as $\mathbb{P}(\text{t11} > t \mid \text{t21} = 5)$, are obtained by differentiating equation (4.1) with respect to the survival margin on which the probability is conditioned. An example is displayed in Figure 4.6.

The insights derived from the copula model are crucial for both clinicians and patients, as individuals with both eyes progressing to late-stage AMD may lose their ability to live independently. In this context, joint progression-free probabilities can help identify patient profiles at high risk. When one eye has already progressed to late-stage AMD, the conditional

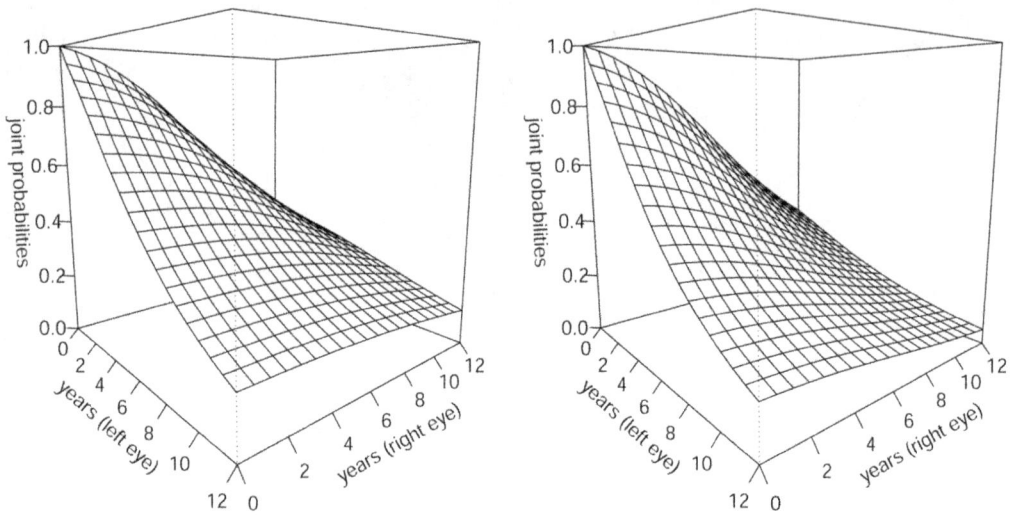

FIGURE 4.5 Joint progression-free probabilities of the left and right eyes for a typical individual, obtained by fitting to the `areds` data a Plackett survival additive distributional regression model with `-logit` margins (left plot), and when assuming that the two margins are not associated (right plot).

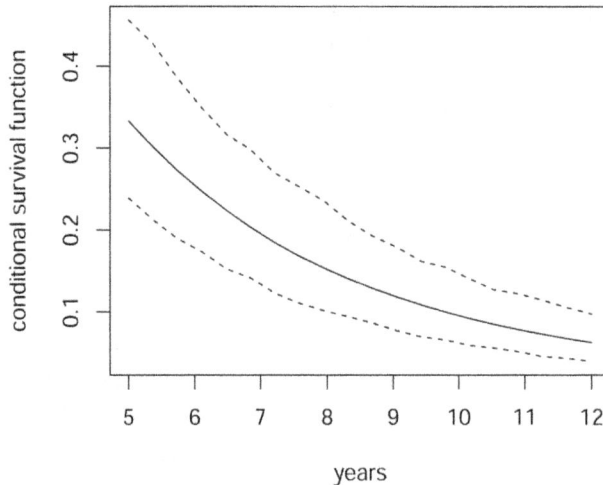

FIGURE 4.6 Estimated progression-free probabilities (with associated 95% intervals) for the left eye of a typical individual conditonal on late-stage AMD disease at 5 years in the right eye, derived from a Plackett survival additive distributional regression model with `-logit` margins fitted to the `areds` data.

progression-free probability for the unaffected eye provides valuable information that can guide efforts to preserve vision in the remaining eye.

The R codes used to produce the plots in Figures 4.2, 4.3, 4.5 and 4.6 are available on the authors' websites.

5

Binary outcomes

Research across numerous domains frequently involves binary outcomes. In public health, malnutrition in children is often assessed using anthropometric indices such as height-for-age and weight-for-age, which are modeled jointly to provide a more coherent and comprehensive risk assessment [Bhuyan et al., 2018]. Another application is found in studies on psychopathology and health service utilization in children, where the responses are binary indicators of borderline clinical mental illness [Horton and Fitzmaurice, 2002]. A further example is provided by Chakraborty et al. [2005], where the goal is to model prostate cancer data to predict the joint probabilities of features indicative of non-organ-confined cancer, such as margin positivity and seminal vesicle positivity.

The copula regression approach by Radice et al. [2016] is discussed and applied to model adverse birth outcomes, specifically low birth weight and preterm birth, highlighting the value of joint modeling in achieving a more nuanced assessment and interpretation of patterns in these responses.

5.1 Adverse birth study

The modeling framework is illustrated using individual-level infant data from 20,000 randomly selected births of female babies in North Carolina in 2008. The aim is to study the association between low birth weight and preterm birth, and how these responses are influenced by various variables. A similar study was conducted by Neelon et al. [2014]. The dataset provides county-level information on maternal characteristics, as well as on the infant birth outcomes of interest (`lbw` = 1 if birth weight is less than 2,500 grams, and `ptb` = 1 if gestational age is less than 37 completed weeks).

Joint regression analysis of `lbw` and `ptb` is essential due to the inherent association between these outcomes, offering a more comprehensive understanding of how maternal and delivery characteristics affect both indicators simultaneously. By accounting for potential synergistic effects and recognizing that infants born both preterm and with low birth weight face compounded health risks, simultaneous modeling offers a more realistic evaluation of high-risk populations.

5.2 Model

The focus is on a pair of binary random variables (Y_1, Y_2), where $Y_j \sim \text{Ber}(\mu_j)$ with $g_{\mu_j}(\mu_j) = \eta_{\mu_j}(\boldsymbol{x}_{\mu_j}; \boldsymbol{\beta}_{\mu_j})$, for $j = 1, 2$. Let $F_j(y_j; \mu_j)$ denote the CDF of Y_j. Using a copula

DOI: 10.1201/9781003593195-5

function $C(\cdot, \cdot; \theta)$, where $g_\theta(\theta) = \eta_\theta(\boldsymbol{x}_\theta; \boldsymbol{\beta}_\theta)$, the probability of $(Y_1 = 1, Y_2 = 1)$ is

$$\mathbb{P}(Y_1 = 1, Y_2 = 1) = C(F_1(1; \mu_1), F_2(1; \mu_2); \theta). \tag{5.1}$$

5.3 Log-likelihood

For a random sample $(y_{i1}, y_{i2}, \boldsymbol{x}_i)_{i=1}^n$, where the covariate vector $\boldsymbol{x}_i$ is the union of $\boldsymbol{x}_{i\mu_1}$, $\boldsymbol{x}_{i\mu_2}$ and $\boldsymbol{x}_{i\theta}$, the log-likelihood function of the binary copula regression model is

$$
\begin{aligned}
\ell(\boldsymbol{\beta}) = \sum_{i=1}^n \{ &y_{i1} y_{i2} \log C(F_1(1; \mu_{i1}), F_2(1; \mu_{i2}); \theta_i) \\
&+ y_{i1}(1 - y_{i2}) \log[F_1(1; \mu_{i1}) - C(F_1(1; \mu_{i1}), F_2(1; \mu_{i2}); \theta_i)] \\
&+ (1 - y_{i1}) y_{i2} \log[F_2(1; \mu_{i2}) - C(F_1(1; \mu_{i1}), F_2(1; \mu_{i2}); \theta_i)] \\
&+ (1 - y_{i1})(1 - y_{i2}) \log[1 - F_1(1; \mu_{i1}) - F_2(1; \mu_{i2}) \\
&+ C(F_1(1; \mu_{i1}), F_2(1; \mu_{i2}); \theta_i)] \}
\end{aligned}
\tag{5.2}
$$

where $\boldsymbol{\beta} = (\boldsymbol{\beta}_{\mu_1}^\top, \boldsymbol{\beta}_{\mu_2}^\top, \boldsymbol{\beta}_\theta^\top)^\top$ is the overall regression coefficient vector.

5.4 Model fitting

Various specifications for the copula (beginning with the Gaussian) and link functions for $g_{\mu_1}(\cdot)$ and $g_{\mu_2}(\cdot)$ were explored. The most supported model, based on convergence checks, parsimony and information-based criteria, uses `probit` link functions and a Gaussian copula with correlation parameter estimated without accounting for covariate effects. The impacts of `age` are modeled flexibly, while geographic effects are incorporated using Gaussian Markov random field smooths, with county boundaries defined in `NC.polys`, a list of polygon vertices delineating North Carolina's counties. In `eq1`, the reduced-rank version of the `mrf` smooth is used, as its *edf* (equal to 10.2) is very close to that of the full-rank version (*edf* = 11). This justifies adopting a model specification with fewer parameters, achieving parsimony without compromising model fit.

```
library(GJRM); library(GJRM.data)
data(infants)
data(NC.polys); xt <- list(polys = NC.polys)

eq1 <- lbw ~ ethnicity + educ + firstbirth + marital + smoke + s(age) +
             s(county, bs = "mrf", xt = xt, k = 50)
eq2 <- ptb ~ ethnicity + educ + firstbirth + marital + smoke + s(age) +
             s(county, bs = "mrf", xt = xt)
fl  <- list(eq1, eq2)

out <- gjrm(fl, margins = c("probit", "probit"), copula = "N",
            model = "B", data = infants)
```

```
conv.check(out)

##
## Maximum absolute gradient value: 2.654232e-10
## Observed information matrix is positive definite
```

Convergence checks are satisfactory, while the findings are summarized in the subsequent outputs and commentary.

```
summary(out)

##
## COPULA: Gaussian
## MARGIN 1: Bernoulli
## MARGIN 2: Bernoulli
##
## EQUATION 1
## Link function for mu1: probit
## Formula: lbw ~ ethnicity + educ + firstbirth + marital + smoke + s(age) +
##     s(county, bs = "mrf", xt = xt, k = 50)
##
## Parametric coefficients:
##                     Estimate Std. Error z value Pr(>|z|)
## (Intercept)         -1.58160    0.09164 -17.259  < 2e-16 ***
## ethnicityHispanic   -0.03575    0.04787  -0.747  0.45521
## ethnicityBlack       0.37493    0.03391  11.055  < 2e-16 ***
## ethnicityOther       0.24623    0.06312   3.901 9.58e-05 ***
## educSecondary        0.02476    0.08689   0.285  0.77572
## educTertiary        -0.07943    0.09014  -0.881  0.37822
## firstbirth           0.12818    0.02957   4.335 1.46e-05 ***
## marital             -0.08801    0.03302  -2.666  0.00768 **
## smoke                0.42552    0.04044  10.522  < 2e-16 ***
## ---
## Signif. codes:  0 '***' 0.001 '**' 0.01 '*' 0.05 '.' 0.1 ' ' 1
##
## Approximate significance of smooth terms:
##              edf Ref.df Chi.sq p-value
## s(age)     2.684   3.39  11.52  0.0142 *
## s(county) 10.199  49.00  14.95  0.0433 *
## ---
## Signif. codes:  0 '***' 0.001 '**' 0.01 '*' 0.05 '.' 0.1 ' ' 1
##
##
## EQUATION 2
## Link function for mu2: probit
## Formula: ptb ~ ethnicity + educ + firstbirth + marital + smoke + s(age) +
##     s(county, bs = "mrf", xt = xt)
##
## Parametric coefficients:
##                     Estimate Std. Error z value Pr(>|z|)
## (Intercept)        -1.242165   0.078232 -15.878  < 2e-16 ***
## ethnicityHispanic  -0.026586   0.042180  -0.630  0.52850
```

```
## ethnicityBlack      0.283113    0.031796    8.904  < 2e-16 ***
## ethnicityOther      0.122551    0.060387    2.029  0.04241 *
## educSecondary      -0.029030    0.073734   -0.394  0.69380
## educTertiary       -0.118289    0.077016   -1.536  0.12457
## firstbirth         -0.009649    0.027470   -0.351  0.72541
## marital            -0.085903    0.030344   -2.831  0.00464 **
## smoke               0.163339    0.039819    4.102  4.1e-05 ***
## ---
## Signif. codes:  0 '***' 0.001 '**' 0.01 '*' 0.05 '.' 0.1 ' ' 1
##
## Approximate significance of smooth terms:
##             edf Ref.df Chi.sq  p-value
## s(age)     4.162  5.157  20.38  0.00118 **
## s(county) 25.706 99.000  52.79 5.69e-06 ***
## ---
## Signif. codes:  0 '***' 0.001 '**' 0.01 '*' 0.05 '.' 0.1 ' ' 1
##
##
## theta = 0.736(0.718,0.757)
## n = 20000   total edf = 61.8
```

As expected, maternal smoking has a significant negative impact on the birth outcomes, being a well-established determinant adversely affecting fetal development. The analysis also reveals that babies born to non-White mothers have a higher likelihood of both lbw and ptb compared to those born to White mothers, highlighting potential ethnic disparities. Being married is associated with a lower risk of adverse birth outcomes, likely reflecting the benefits of marital stability and related socioeconomic advantages that contribute to improved prenatal care. In contrast, first births are associated with a higher probability of low birth weight, possibly due to the uterus and placenta adapting for the first time and increased maternal stress.

```
par(mfrow = c(1, 2))
plot(out, eq = 1, select = 1, scale = 0)
plot(out, eq = 2, select = 1, scale = 0)

par(mfrow = c(2, 1))
plot(out, eq = 1, select = 2, scheme = 1)
plot(out, eq = 2, select = 2, scheme = 1)
```

The plots in Figures 5.1 and 5.2 provide a detailed visualization of the effects of age and county. Older maternal age is associated with a higher likelihood of low birth weight. Geographically, the risk of lbw is lower in western North Carolina, suggesting regional variations that may be linked to local healthcare access and socioeconomic conditions. The risk of ptb is higher for both younger and older mothers. Moreover, the risk of preterm birth is lower in some of the northeastern regions of North Carolina, potentially reflecting better prenatal care or more favorable conditions in these areas.

The estimated copula parameter reveals a relatively strong correlation between the outcomes, after accounting for observed covariates, suggesting that variables, such as genetic predispositions and environmental exposures, are likely influencing both lbw and ptb.

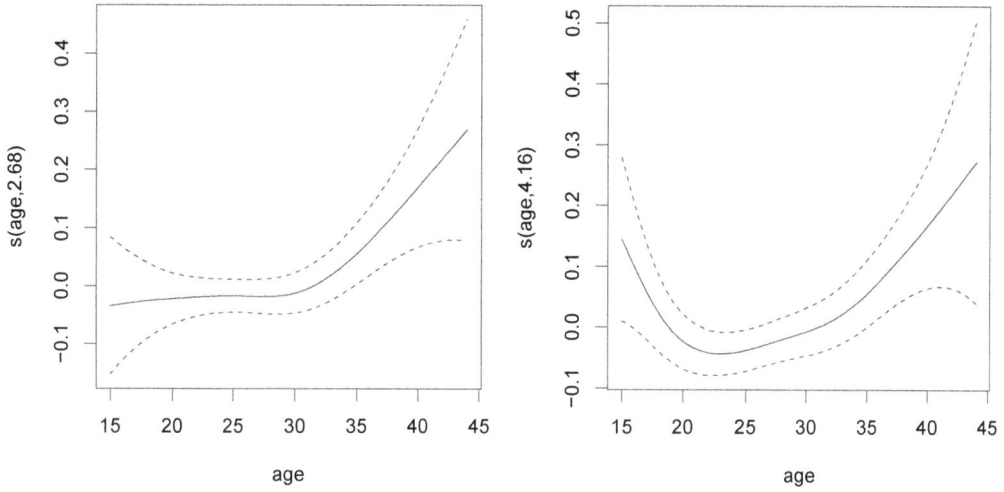

FIGURE 5.1 Estimated effects (with associated 95% intervals) of `age` on the scales of the additive predictors of μ_1 and μ_2, derived from a bivariate probit model fitted to the `infants` data.

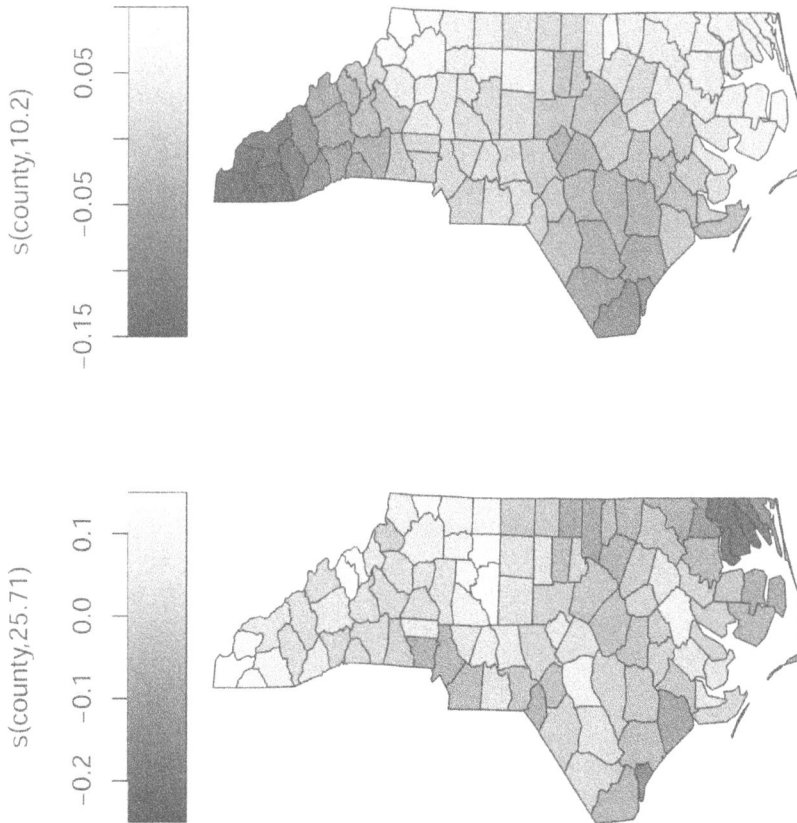

FIGURE 5.2 Estimated effects of `county` on the scales of the additive predictors of μ_1 and μ_2, derived from a bivariate probit model fitted to the `infants` data.

Marginal probabilities for a typical female infant being preterm or having a low birth weight are obtained as follows.

```
nd <- data.frame(ethnicity = "White", educ = "Tertiary", county = 60,
                 firstbirth = 0, marital = 1, smoke = 0, age = 26)
marg.mv(out, eq = 1, newdata = nd)
```

```
##
## Marginal mean with 95% interval:
##
## 0.0391 (0.0343,0.0485)
```

```
marg.mv(out, eq = 2, newdata = nd)
```

```
##
## Marginal mean with 95% interval:
##
## 0.0623 (0.0539,0.0713)
```

The results reveal a 3.9% likelihood of preterm delivery and a 6.2% probability of low birth weight. While these outcomes are relatively uncommon, the risk of low birth weight appears slightly higher than that of preterm birth for an infant with these characteristics.

Joint probabilities, such as $\mathbb{P}(\text{lbw} = 1, \text{ptb} = 1)$, are calculated using (5.1).

```
lr <- length(NC.polys); res.BYc <- NA

for(i in 1:lr){
   nd$county <- i
   res.BYc[i] <- copula.prob(out, y1 = 1, y2 = 1, newdata = nd)$p12*100
             }
polys.map(NC.polys, res.BYc, scheme = "gray")
```

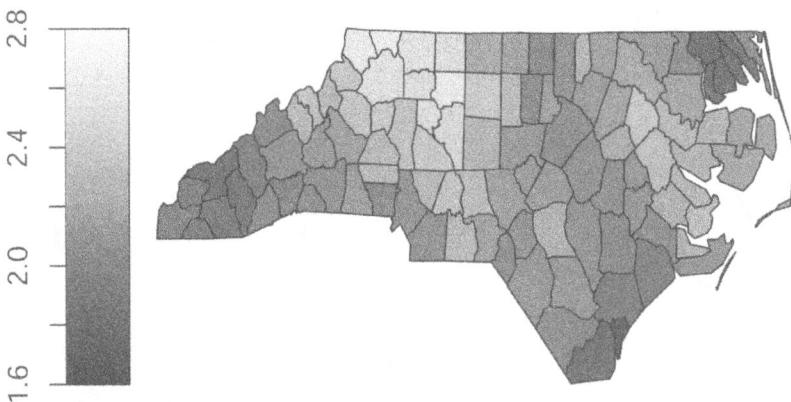

FIGURE 5.3 Joint probabilities (expressed as percentages) of experiencing both adverse outcomes for a typical female infant by `county`, derived from a bivariate probit model fitted to the `infants` data.

Figure 5.3 illustrates that the risk (in %) of a typical female infant being both preterm and low birth weight varies across counties, with Ashe, Alleghany, Surry and Wilkes exhibiting the highest joint probabilities.

Conditional probabilities, such as $\mathbb{P}(\texttt{lbw} = 1|\texttt{ptb} = 1)$, may also be of interest and are computed as the ratio between (5.1) and the marginal CDF on which the probability is conditioned.

```
nd$county <- 60 # typical county
copula.prob(out, y1 = 1, y2 = 1, cond = 2, newdata = nd, intervals = TRUE)
```

```
##           p12       2.5%      97.5%
##    0.3305712 0.292749 0.3748229
```

```
copula.prob(out, y1 = 1, y2 = 1, cond = 2, newdata = nd, intervals = TRUE,
            joint = FALSE)
```

```
##            p12        2.5%      97.5%
##    0.03957563 0.03416617 0.04634998
```

The estimates suggest that given an infant is preterm, the probability of also being low birth weight is 33% according to the copula model, compared to 4% under the assumption of independence between the two outcomes. This emphasizes the need for an approach that accounts for the inherent association between the responses, leading to more realistic and coherent risk assessments.

Figure 5.4, produced using the R code available on the authors' websites, shows the joint probabilities of experiencing both adverse outcomes for a typical female infant of a smoking mother by county. As expected, the risks are higher than those for an infant of a non-smoking mother, displayed in Figure 5.3.

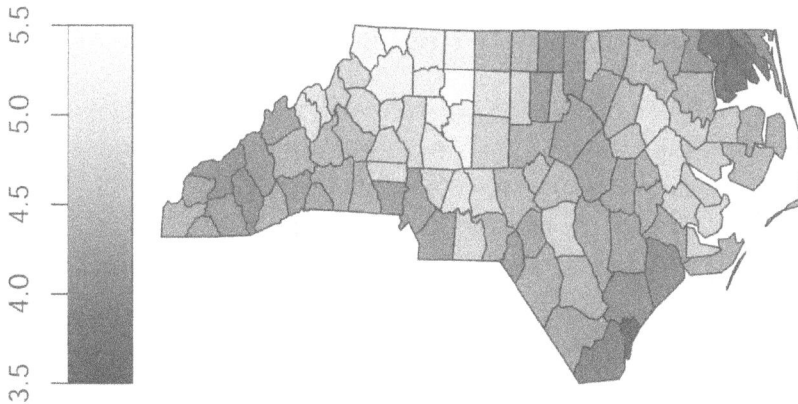

FIGURE 5.4 Joint probabilities (expressed as percentages) of experiencing both adverse outcomes for a typical female infant of a smoking mother by `county`, derived from a bivariate probit model fitted to the `infants` data.

5.5 Trivariate extension

Although this book primarily addresses bivariate responses, for the case of binary outcomes, GJRM supports the specification of a trivariate additive regression model. Let (Y_1, Y_2, Y_3) be a triplet of binary random variables. The probability of $(Y_1 = 1, Y_2 = 1, Y_3 = 1)$ is defined as

$$\mathbb{P}(Y_1 = 1, Y_2 = 1, Y_3 = 1) = \Phi_3 \left(\Phi^{-1}\{F_1(1; \mu_1)\}, \Phi^{-1}\{F_2(1; \mu_2)\}, \Phi^{-1}\{F_3(1; \mu_3)\}; \mathbf{\Sigma} \right),$$
(5.3)

where $F_j(1; \mu_j)$ with $g_{\mu_j}(\mu_j) = \eta_{\mu_j}(\boldsymbol{x}_{\mu_j}; \boldsymbol{\beta}_{\mu_j})$, for $j = 1, 2, 3$, denotes the CDF of Y_j and $\Phi_3(\cdot, \cdot, \cdot; \cdot)$ is the CDF of a standard trivariate Gaussian distribution with dependence parameters $g_{\theta_{12}}(\theta_{12}) = \eta_{\theta_{12}}(\boldsymbol{x}_{\theta_{12}}; \boldsymbol{\beta}_{\theta_{12}})$, $g_{\theta_{13}}(\theta_{13}) = \eta_{\theta_{13}}(\boldsymbol{x}_{\theta_{13}}; \boldsymbol{\beta}_{\theta_{13}})$ and $g_{\theta_{23}}(\theta_{23}) = \eta_{\theta_{23}}(\boldsymbol{x}_{\theta_{23}}; \boldsymbol{\beta}_{\theta_{23}})$. The matrix $\mathbf{\Sigma}$ is equal to

$$\mathbf{\Sigma} = \begin{pmatrix} 1 & \theta_{12} & \theta_{13} \\ \theta_{12} & 1 & \theta_{23} \\ \theta_{13} & \theta_{23} & 1 \end{pmatrix},$$

where $\theta_{jj'}$ is the correlation coefficient between the jth and j'^{th} outcomes for $j = 1, 2$ and $j' = 2, 3$ with $j \neq j'$. Positive-definiteness of $\mathbf{\Sigma}$ is imposed using the methods discussed in Filippou et al. [2017] and [2019].

The case of non-Gaussian dependence has not been developed yet. However, as observed by Filippou et al. [2019] in simulation studies, the Gaussian copula generally appears to be a sensible and tractable modeling choice for binary outcomes.

For a random sample $(y_{i1}, y_{i2}, y_{i3}, \boldsymbol{x}_i)_{i=1}^n$, where the covariate vector $\boldsymbol{x}_i$ is the union of $\boldsymbol{x}_{i\mu_1}$, $\boldsymbol{x}_{i\mu_2}$, $\boldsymbol{x}_{i\mu_3}$, $\boldsymbol{x}_{i\theta_{12}}$, $\boldsymbol{x}_{i\theta_{13}}$ and $\boldsymbol{x}_{i\theta_{23}}$, the log-likelihood function of the trivariate binary copula model is

$$
\begin{aligned}
\ell(\boldsymbol{\beta}) = \sum_{i=1}^n \{ & y_{i1}y_{i2}y_{i3}\log(p_{i123}) + (1 - y_{i1})y_{i2}y_{i3}\log(p_{i23} - p_{i123}) \\
& + y_{i1}(1 - y_{i2})y_{i3}\log(p_{i13} - p_{i123}) + y_{i1}y_{i2}(1 - y_{i3})\log(p_{i12} - p_{i123}) \\
& + y_{i1}(1 - y_{i2})(1 - y_{i3})\log(p_{i1} - p_{i12} - p_{i13} + p_{i123}) \\
& + (1 - y_{i1})y_{i2}(1 - y_{i3})\log(p_{i2} - p_{i12} - p_{i23} + p_{i123}) \\
& + (1 - y_{i1})(1 - y_{i2})y_{i3}\log(p_{i3} - p_{i23} - p_{i13} + p_{i123}) \\
& + (1 - y_{i1})(1 - y_{i2})(1 - y_{i3})\log(1 - p_{i1} - p_{i2} - p_{i3} + p_{i12} + p_{i23} + p_{i13} - p_{i123}) \},
\end{aligned}
$$

where $\boldsymbol{\beta} = (\boldsymbol{\beta}_{\mu_1}^\top, \boldsymbol{\beta}_{\mu_2}^\top, \boldsymbol{\beta}_{\mu_3}^\top, \boldsymbol{\beta}_{\theta_{12}}^\top, \boldsymbol{\beta}_{\theta_{13}}^\top, \boldsymbol{\beta}_{\theta_{23}}^\top)^\top$ is the overall regression coefficient vector, p_{123} is equal to (5.3), $p_{jj'} = \Phi_2(F_j(1; \mu_j), F_{j'}(1; \mu_{j'}); \theta_{jj'})$ for $j = 1, 2$ and $j' = 2, 3$, with $j \neq j'$, and $p_j = F_j(1; \mu_j)$ for $j = 1, 2, 3$.

The trivariate extension could be used to jointly model three adverse birth outcomes such as low birth weight, preterm birth and neonatal intensive care unit admission. Section 12.5 discusses another possible application.

6

Ordinal outcomes

Models for bivariate ordinal responses can address a range of empirical challenges. For example, Donat and Marra [2018] applied copula regression to the study of road accidents, while Weiss [1993], Card and Giuliano [2013] and Imai et al. [2023] explored related approaches in contexts such as road safety, social interactions and risky behaviors, and the pretrial Public Safety Assessment in the U.S. criminal justice system, respectively.

This chapter applies the method introduced by Donat and Marra [2018] to examine both general and mental health perceptions, providing insights into the relationship between these outcomes and the variables influencing them. Moreover, predictions generated by the joint model provide meaningful perspectives on health perceptions across various scenarios.

6.1 Perceived health

The case study utilizes the MEPS data introduced in Chapter 3. The outcomes of interest, `general` and `mental` (representing perceived general and mental health), are rated on a scale from 1 to 5 (excellent = 1, very good = 2, good = 3, fair = 4, poor = 5). The available regressors are `bmi`, `income`, `age`, `gender`, `ethnicity`, `education`, `region`, `hypertension` and `hyperlipidemia`.

Joint modeling captures the interplay between physical and mental health, acknowledging that a poor perception of physical health can negatively impact mental well-being (e.g., leading to anxiety or depression) and vice versa. Furthermore, insights from the simultaneous model can inform more effective interventions and policies, fostering the development of integrated strategies that address both aspects of wellness simultaneously.

6.2 Model

Consider a pair of ordinal variables (Y_1, Y_2). Each of them is defined as

$$
Y_j = \begin{cases}
1 & \text{if} \quad Y_j^* \leq c_{j1} \\
2 & \text{if} \quad c_{j1} < Y_j^* \leq c_{j2} \\
\vdots & \\
k_j & \text{if} \quad c_{jk_j-1} < Y_j^* \leq c_{jk_j} \\
\vdots & \\
K_j & \text{if} \quad c_{jK_j-1} < Y_j^* \leq c_{jK_j}
\end{cases} \quad , \quad j = 1, 2 \,,
$$

DOI: 10.1201/9781003593195-6

where $Y_j^* \sim D_j(\mu_j, \sigma_j)$ and $D_j(\cdot, \cdot)$ is either a Gaussian or logistic distribution with $g_{\mu_j}(\mu_j) = \eta_{\mu_j}(\boldsymbol{x}_{\mu_j}; \boldsymbol{\beta}_{\mu_j})$ and $\sigma_j = 1$. The unknown cutoff points $c_{j1}, c_{j2}, \ldots, c_{jK_j-1}$ are real numbers that satisfy the monotonic condition $-\infty = c_{j0} < c_{j1} < c_{j2} < \cdots < c_{jK_j-1} < c_{jK_j} = \infty$.

The joint probability of $Y_1 = k_1$ and $Y_2 = k_2$ is given by

$$
\begin{aligned}
\mathbb{P}(Y_1 = k_1, Y_2 = k_2) &= \mathbb{P}(c_{1k_1-1} < Y_1^* \le c_{1k_1}, c_{2k_2-1} < Y_2^* \le c_{2k_2}) \\
&= \mathbb{P}(Y_1^* \le c_{1k_1}, Y_2^* \le c_{2k_2}) - \mathbb{P}(Y_1^* \le c_{1k_1-1}, Y_2^* \le c_{2k_2}) \\
&\quad - \mathbb{P}(Y_1^* \le c_{1k_1}, Y_2^* \le c_{2k_2-1}) + \mathbb{P}(Y_1^* \le c_{1k_1-1}, Y_2^* \le c_{2k_2-1})
\end{aligned} \tag{6.1}
$$

Using a copula function $C(\cdot, \cdot; \theta)$, where $g_\theta(\theta) = \eta_\theta(\boldsymbol{x}_\theta; \boldsymbol{\beta}_\theta)$, equation (6.1) can be expressed as

$$
\begin{aligned}
\mathbb{P}(Y_1 = k_1, Y_2 = k_2) = \ & C(F_1(c_{1k_1} - \mu_1), F_2(c_{2k_2} - \mu_2); \theta) \\
& - C(F_1(c_{1k_1-1} - \mu_1), F_2(c_{2k_2} - \mu_2); \theta) \\
& - C(F_1(c_{1k_1} - \mu_1), F_2(c_{2k_2-1} - \mu_2); \theta) \\
& + C(F_1(c_{1k_1-1} - \mu_1), F_2(c_{2k_2-1} - \mu_2); \theta)
\end{aligned} \tag{6.2}
$$

where $F_j(\cdot)$ denotes the jth CDF of either a standard Gaussian or standard logistic distribution.

6.3   Log-likelihood

Using equation (6.2), for a random sample $(y_{i1}, y_{i2}, \boldsymbol{x}_i)_{i=1}^n$, where the covariate vector $\boldsymbol{x}_i$ is the union of $\boldsymbol{x}_{i\mu_1}$, $\boldsymbol{x}_{i\mu_2}$ and $\boldsymbol{x}_{i\theta}$, the log-likelihood of the ordinal copula regression model is

$$
\begin{aligned}
\ell(\boldsymbol{\beta}) = \sum_{i=1}^n \sum_{k_1=1}^{K_1} \sum_{k_2=1}^{K_2} & \mathbb{1}_{y_{i1}=k_1, y_{i2}=k_2} \log \{ C(F_1(c_{1k_1} - \mu_{i1}), F_2(c_{2k_2} - \mu_{i2}); \theta_i) \\
& - C(F_1(c_{1k_1-1} - \mu_{i1}), F_2(c_{2k_2} - \mu_{i2}); \theta_i) - C(F_1(c_{1k_1} - \mu_{i1}), F_2(c_{2k_2-1} - \mu_{i2}); \theta_i) \\
& + C(F_1(c_{1k_1-1} - \mu_{i1}), F_2(c_{2k_2-1} - \mu_{i2}); \theta_i) \}
\end{aligned}
$$

where $\boldsymbol{\beta} = (\boldsymbol{c}_1^\top, \boldsymbol{c}_2^\top, \boldsymbol{\beta}_{\mu_1}^\top, \boldsymbol{\beta}_{\mu_2}^\top, \boldsymbol{\beta}_\theta^\top)^\top$ is the overall parameter vector, with $\boldsymbol{c}_1$ and $\boldsymbol{c}_2$ including all the cutoff parameters for the two equations.

6.4   Model fitting

The equations for μ_1, μ_2 and θ are specified as

```
library(GJRM); library(GJRM.data)
data(meps)
eq1 <- general ~ s(bmi) + s(income) + s(age) + s(education) + ethnicity +
                 region + gender + hypertension + hyperlipidemia
eq2 <- mental  ~ s(bmi) + s(income) + s(age) + s(education) + ethnicity +
                 region + gender + hypertension + hyperlipidemia
eq3 <-         ~ s(bmi) + s(income) + s(age) + s(education) + ethnicity +
                 region + gender + hypertension + hyperlipidemia
```

The options for the margins are the standard Gaussian and logistic distributions. For the dependence structure, a Gaussian copula is considered initially, followed by alternative copulae that are consistent with the sign and strength of the observed correlation. Based on convergence and information-based criteria, as well as considerations of parsimony, the preferred model is

```
out  <- gjrm(list(eq1, eq2, eq3), data = meps,
            margins = c("ord.logit", "ord.logit"), copula = "PL",
            model = "B", uni.fit = TRUE)
conv.check(out)
```

```
##
## Maximum absolute gradient value: 2.967404e-11
## Observed information matrix is positive definite
```

Convergence checks are satisfactory, while the results are summarized thereafter.

```
summary(out)
```

```
##
## COPULA: Plackett
## MARGIN 1: Ordinal
## MARGIN 2: Ordinal
##
## EQUATION 1
## Link function for mu1: logit
## Formula: general ~ s(bmi) + s(income) + s(age) + s(education) + ethnicity
##      + region + gender + hypertension + hyperlipidemia
##
## Parametric coefficients:
##                 Estimate Std. Error z value Pr(>|z|)
## ethnicity2      -0.22906    0.04625  -4.953 7.33e-07 ***
## ethnicity3      -0.06981    0.19100  -0.365   0.7148
## ethnicity4      -0.03969    0.06476  -0.613   0.5400
## region2          0.10060    0.05969   1.685   0.0919 .
## region3         -0.04063    0.05325  -0.763   0.4454
## region4          0.02715    0.05676   0.478   0.6324
## gender          -0.22751    0.03563  -6.386 1.70e-10 ***
## hypertension     0.67524    0.04778  14.131  < 2e-16 ***
## hyperlipidemia   0.57512    0.04810  11.956  < 2e-16 ***
## ---
## Signif. codes:  0 '***' 0.001 '**' 0.01 '*' 0.05 '.' 0.1 ' ' 1
##
## Approximate significance of smooth terms:
##                 edf Ref.df Chi.sq p-value
## s(bmi)        4.798  5.828  245.2  <2e-16 ***
## s(income)     6.285  7.358  287.4  <2e-16 ***
## s(age)        3.791  4.684  220.1  <2e-16 ***
## s(education)  4.548  5.499  158.3  <2e-16 ***
## ---
## Signif. codes:  0 '***' 0.001 '**' 0.01 '*' 0.05 '.' 0.1 ' ' 1
##
##
```

```
## EQUATION 2
## Link function for mu2: logit
## Formula: mental ~ s(bmi) + s(income) + s(age) + s(education) + ethnicity
##     + region + gender + hypertension + hyperlipidemia
##
## Parametric coefficients:
##                 Estimate Std. Error z value Pr(>|z|)
## ethnicity2      -0.21174    0.04651  -4.552 5.31e-06 ***
## ethnicity3       0.13749    0.19228   0.715 0.474578
## ethnicity4      -0.14169    0.06542  -2.166 0.030322 *
## region2          0.04374    0.05961   0.734 0.463084
## region3         -0.22754    0.05320  -4.277 1.89e-05 ***
## region4         -0.16846    0.05669  -2.972 0.002961 **
## gender          -0.13382    0.03571  -3.747 0.000179 ***
## hypertension     0.44149    0.04756   9.283  < 2e-16 ***
## hyperlipidemia   0.39601    0.04782   8.281  < 2e-16 ***
## ---
## Signif. codes:  0 '***' 0.001 '**' 0.01 '*' 0.05 '.' 0.1 ' ' 1
##
## Approximate significance of smooth terms:
##               edf Ref.df Chi.sq p-value
## s(bmi)      4.468  5.462  74.81  <2e-16 ***
## s(income)   6.295  7.368 225.27  <2e-16 ***
## s(age)      3.144  3.905 138.53  <2e-16 ***
## s(education) 4.039 4.936 128.52  <2e-16 ***
## ---
## Signif. codes:  0 '***' 0.001 '**' 0.01 '*' 0.05 '.' 0.1 ' ' 1
##
##
## EQUATION 3
## Link function for theta: log
## Formula: ~s(bmi) + s(income) + s(age) + s(education) + ethnicity + region
##     + gender + hypertension + hyperlipidemia
##
## Parametric coefficients:
##                 Estimate Std. Error z value Pr(>|z|)
## (Intercept)      3.01181    0.10352  29.094  < 2e-16 ***
## ethnicity2       0.13611    0.09544   1.426  0.15384
## ethnicity3       0.12307    0.41282   0.298  0.76562
## ethnicity4       0.27923    0.14145   1.974  0.04838 *
## region2          0.06264    0.12372   0.506  0.61264
## region3         -0.17313    0.10863  -1.594  0.11102
## region4         -0.06709    0.11734  -0.572  0.56746
## gender           0.23577    0.07363   3.202  0.00136 **
## hypertension    -0.44899    0.09315  -4.820 1.43e-06 ***
## hyperlipidemia  -0.40686    0.09387  -4.334 1.46e-05 ***
## ---
## Signif. codes:  0 '***' 0.001 '**' 0.01 '*' 0.05 '.' 0.1 ' ' 1
##
## Approximate significance of smooth terms:
##               edf Ref.df Chi.sq p-value
```

```
## s(bmi)       2.817  3.571 19.260 0.00052 ***
## s(income)    1.683  2.108  6.416 0.04718 *
## s(age)       1.852  2.318 19.279 0.00016 ***
## s(education) 2.893  3.614  4.039 0.41847
## ---
## Signif. codes:  0 '***' 0.001 '**' 0.01 '*' 0.05 '.' 0.1 ' ' 1
##
##
## theta = 20.2(15.5,27.2)
## n = 10638  total edf = 82.6
```

Having `hypertension` and `hyperlipidemia` significantly increases the probability of poor perceptions of both general and mental health, aligning with existing medical research showing that chronic illnesses often negatively impact overall well-being. The covariates `ethnicity` and `gender` also significantly impact the responses, most likely due to differences in healthcare access, cultural attitudes toward health, as well as biological and behavioral influences on health perceptions. The `region` variable primarily affects mental health, suggesting an influence of location-related aspects such as the availability of mental health services or local socioeconomic conditions.

```
plot(out, eq = 1, pages = 1, scale = 0, rug = TRUE, jit = TRUE)
```

Figure 6.1 illustrates several key patterns. Firstly, as individuals age, their perception of poor general health tends to increase at varying rates rather than steadily. Secondly, poor general health perception generally declines with `education`. The increase observed at lower education levels is accompanied by wide intervals, indicating substantial uncertainty in this range. Thirdly, the perception of poor general health tends to rise with higher `bmi` values. However, there is also some evidence of an increase at very low `bmi` levels, although the variability is considerable due to the limited number of individuals in this category. Lastly, perceived poor general health decreases with increasing `income`, although this effect levels off when `income` exceeds approximately \$160,000. The results for `mental`, not shown here but reproducible using the same plotting command for `eq = 2`, reveal similar trends.

The copula parameter quantifies the degree of dependence between the perceived health outcomes, likely stemming from unmeasured variables such as lifestyle and social environment. For simplicity of exposition, only lifestyle will be considered a potential influence when interpreting the covariate effects.

If a healthier lifestyle reduces the perception of poor general and mental health (as indicated by the positive sign of the dependence parameter, which is consistent with a negative effect of lifestyle on both outcomes), then such an improvement seems to be greater for males compared to females. Furthermore, the impact of a healthier lifestyle is likely to be less pronounced for individuals with `hypertension` and `hyperlipidemia` as these conditions may limit perceived health improvements despite positive changes in behavior.

```
plot(out, eq = 3, pages = 1, scale = 0, rug = TRUE, jit = TRUE)
```

Figure 6.2 suggests that increases in `bmi` and `age` are associated with a reduced effectiveness of a healthier lifestyle in improving perceived health outcomes. This may be due to comorbidities linked to higher `bmi` as well as age-related physiological changes that hinder the adoption of healthy behaviors. Conversely, higher `income` associates with a greater positive impact of a healthier lifestyle, as individuals with more resources typically have better access to quality food, fitness programs and healthcare services. Education does not appear to have any impact in this case.

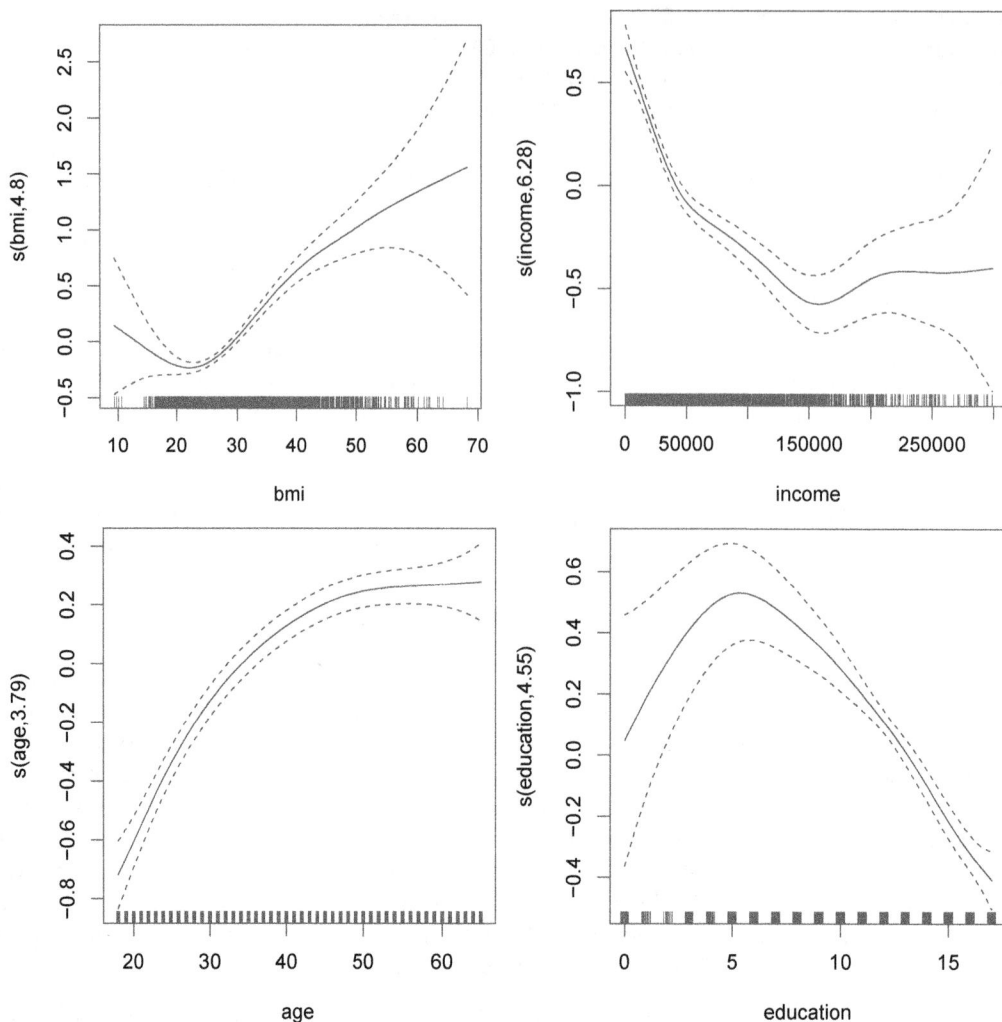

FIGURE 6.1 Estimated smooth effects (with associated 95% intervals) of `bmi`, `income`, `age` and `education` on the scale of the additive predictor of μ_1, derived from a Plackett copula additive distributional regression model with ordinal logit margins fitted to the `meps` data.

These findings highlight the valuable insights offered by the copula additive distributional regression model, which can guide more effective interventions and policies that address multiple aspects of well-being by revealing the complex interplay between responses and covariates.

Joint and conditional probabilities are calculated using (6.2) and the ratio of (6.2) to the marginal PMF on which the probability is conditioned.

```
nd <- data.frame(bmi = 27, income = 47000, age = 40, gender = 0,
                 ethnicity = 1, region = 3, education = 12,
                 hypertension = 0, hyperlipidemia = 0)

copula.prob(out, y1 = 1, y2 = 1, newdata = nd, intervals = TRUE)
```

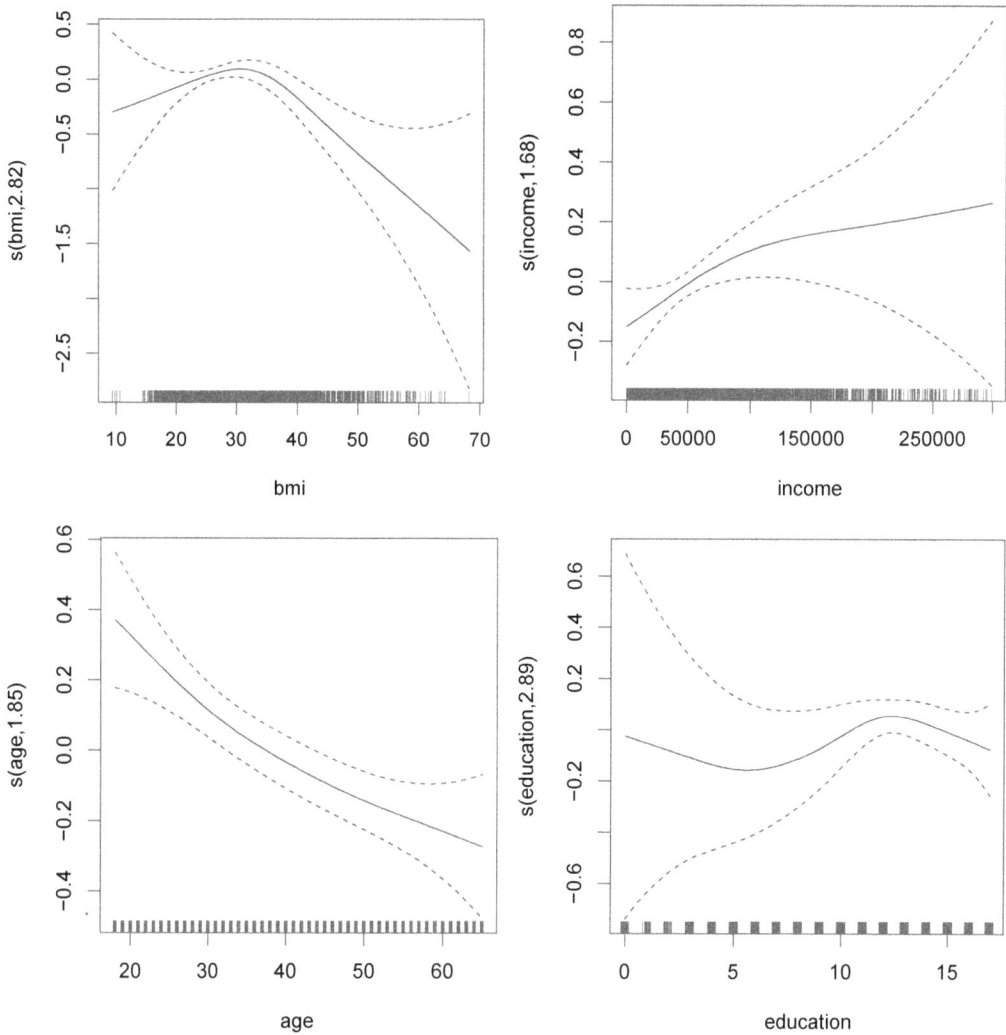

FIGURE 6.2 Estimated smooth effects (with associated 95% intervals) of `bmi`, `income`, `age` and `education` on the scale of the additive predictor of θ, derived from a Plackett copula additive distributional regression model with ordinal logit margins fitted to the `meps` data.

```
##          p12       2.5%      97.5%
##    0.2307638 0.2100965 0.2530576
copula.prob(out, y1 = 1, y2 = 1, newdata = nd, joint = FALSE,
            intervals = TRUE)

##          p12       2.5%      97.5%
##    0.1034741 0.09175673 0.1153018
```

For a representative individual, the copula model estimates the probability of perceiving excellent general and mental health at 0.23, which is significantly higher than the value obtained under the assumption of independence of the outcomes.

```
copula.prob(out, y1 = 1, y2 = 5, newdata = nd, cond = 2, intervals = TRUE)
```

```
##          p12        2.5%        97.5%
##    0.02090158 0.01690556 0.02742962
```

```
copula.prob(out, y1 = 1, y2 = 1, newdata = nd, cond = 2, intervals = TRUE)
```

```
##          p12        2.5%       97.5%
##    0.6038333 0.5714925 0.635168
```

The probability that a typical individual reports their general health as excellent, given that they perceive their mental health as poor, is quite low. In contrast, when this individual rates their mental health as excellent, the likelihood of also rating their general health as excellent is relatively high. Similar patterns emerge when examining the reverse.

7

Binary outcome with partial observability

In certain applications, an observed binary outcome reflects the joint realization of two unobserved binary choices, each determined by a different decision maker. To account for this partial observability, Poirier [1980] introduced a bivariate probit model in which only one of the four possible joint outcomes is observed. The model includes two equations, describing the underlying unobserved responses, which are linked through a bivariate Gaussian distribution, with the correlation coefficient capturing the influence of unmeasured variables affecting both outcomes.

This chapter discusses an extension of the model by Poirier [1980] and uses it to analyze data on civil war onset. Results on covariate effects and joint probabilities are compared with those from a standard probit model, emphasizing the complex interplay between economic variables and political decision-making.

7.1 Civil war onset

To highlight the benefits of using a bivariate probit model with partial observability, the analysis of civil war onset by Fearon and Laitin [2003], as revisited by Nieman [2015], is examined. A civil war is often theorized to result from interactions between an opposition group and the government. As such, only their joint decision (war onset) is observable, rather than the individual decisions. Fearon's study identifies the variables that increase the likelihood of civil war onset, but it does not distinguish between the covariates that drive local populations to rebel and those that motivate governments to engage in conflict.

As in Nieman [2015], the proposed model includes the variables in the `war` data frame, which consists of 6,326 observations. The outcome of interest is `onset`, coded as 1 for all country-years in which a civil war began.

7.2 Model

Let us assume that a binary outcome Y reflects the joint realization of two unobserved binary responses Y_1 and Y_2. It is only possible to observe the product of Y_1 and Y_2. Therefore, $Y = 1$ only if $Y_1 = Y_2 = 1$ and 0 otherwise. As a result, $\mathbb{P}(Y = 1) = \mathbb{P}(Y_1 = 1, Y_2 = 1)$ and $\mathbb{P}(Y = 0) = 1 - \mathbb{P}(Y_1 = 1, Y_2 = 1)$.

For $j = 1, 2$, $Y_j \sim \text{Ber}(\mu_j)$ with $g_{\mu_j}(\mu_j) = \eta_{\mu_j}(\boldsymbol{x}_{\mu_j}; \boldsymbol{\beta}_{\mu_j})$. This implies that $Y \sim \text{Ber}(\mu)$, where $\mu = \mathbb{P}(Y_1 = 1, Y_2 = 1)$. Let $F_j(y_j; \mu_j)$ denote the CDF of Y_j. Using a copula function

$C(\cdot, \cdot; \theta)$,

$$\mathbb{P}(Y = 1) = C(F_1(1; \mu_1), F_2(1; \mu_2); \theta), \tag{7.1}$$

whereas $\mathbb{P}(Y = 0)$ is given by the complement of (7.1).

7.3   Log-likelihood

For a random sample $(y_i, \boldsymbol{x}_i)_{i=1}^n$, where the covariate vector $\boldsymbol{x}_i$ is the union of $\boldsymbol{x}_{i\mu_1}$ and $\boldsymbol{x}_{i\mu_2}$, the log-likelihood function of the binary partial observability model is

$$\ell(\boldsymbol{\beta}) = \sum_{i=1}^n [y_i \log \{C(F_1(1; \mu_{i1}), F_2(1; \mu_{i2}); \theta)\} \\ + (1 - y_i) \log \{1 - C(F_1(1; \mu_{i1}), F_2(1; \mu_{i2}); \theta)\}] \tag{7.2}$$

where $\boldsymbol{\beta} = (\boldsymbol{\beta}_{\mu_1}^\top, \boldsymbol{\beta}_{\mu_2}^\top, \theta)^\top$ is the overall regression coefficient vector.

The model has been shown to be identified under the Gaussian assumption, where equation (7.1) is specified as $C(F_1(1; \mu_{i1}), F_2(1; \mu_{i2}); \theta) = \Phi_2(\eta_{i\mu_1}(\boldsymbol{x}_{i\mu_1}; \boldsymbol{\beta}_{\mu_1}), \eta_{i\mu_2}(\boldsymbol{x}_{i\mu_2}; \boldsymbol{\beta}_{\mu_2}); \theta)$. Furthermore, the nonlinearity of (7.2) ensures local identification of the model parameters, except in specific cases involving unusual configurations of exogenous variables [Poirier, 1980]. When the unobservables influencing both outcomes are not associated, the model can be simplified by setting $\theta = 0$ [Abowd and Farber, 1982]. Since interchanging $\eta_{i\mu_1}(\boldsymbol{x}_{i\mu_1}; \boldsymbol{\beta}_{\mu_1})$ and $\eta_{i\mu_2}(\boldsymbol{x}_{i\mu_2}; \boldsymbol{\beta}_{\mu_2})$ would result in an observationally equivalent model (a situation Poirier terms the labeling problem), the equations for the two underlying responses are typically distinguished by imposing at least one exclusion restriction on the covariates.

7.4   Model fitting

The starting model is

```
library(GJRM); library(GJRM.data)
data(war)

reb.eq <- onset ~ instab + oil + cwar + lpop + lmnt + ethfrac + poldem +
                  s(gdp) + s(relfrac)
gov.eq <- onset ~ instab + oil + cwar + ncontig + nwstate + s(gdp)
fl     <- list(reb.eq, gov.eq)

bpo <- gjrm(fl, margins = c("probit", "probit"), model = "BPO", data = war)
conv.check(bpo)
```

```
##
## Maximum absolute gradient value: 0.3306975
## Observed information matrix is positive definite
```

```
c(bpo$edf[[1]], bpo$edf[[2]])
```

```
##      s(gdp)  s(relfrac)       s(gdp)
##           1           1            1
summary(bpo)
```

```
...
##
## theta = 0.0546(-0.818,0.942)
...
```

The convergence diagnostics suggest that the model may be overly complex. The estimated smooth functions have *edf* = 1, indicating that the effects of `gdp` and `relfrac` are linear on the scale of the respective additive predictors. Moreover, the estimate for θ and its interval point to a lack of correlation between the responses. Consequently, the model can be simplified by setting $\theta = 0$ and modeling the impacts of `gdp` and `relfrac` linearly.

```
reb.eq <- onset ~ instab + oil + cwar + lpop + lmnt + ethfrac + poldem +
                  gdp + relfrac
gov.eq <- onset ~ instab + oil + cwar + ncontig + nwstate + gdp
fl     <- list(reb.eq, gov.eq)

bpo0 <- gjrm(fl, margins = c("probit", "probit"),
             model = "BPO0", data = war)
conv.check(bpo0)
```

```
##
## Maximum absolute gradient value: 1.523718e-06
## Observed information matrix is positive definite
```

For comparison, using `mgcv`, a univariate probit model is also fitted. Here, the combined outcomes of opposition groups and governments are modeled without distinguishing between their individual decisions.

```
library(mgcv)
```

```
## Loading required package: nlme
```

```
## This is mgcv 1.9-1. For overview type 'help("mgcv-package")'.
war.eq <- onset ~ instab + oil + cwar + ncontig + nwstate + lpop + lmnt +
                  ethfrac + poldem + gdp + relfrac
pb <- gam(war.eq, family = binomial(link = "probit"), data = war)

summary(bpo0)
```

```
##
## COPULA: Gaussian
## MARGIN 1: Bernoulli
## MARGIN 2: Bernoulli
##
## EQUATION 1
## Link function for mu1: probit
```

```
## Formula: onset ~ instab + oil + cwar + lpop + lmnt + ethfrac + poldem +
##     gdp + relfrac
##
## Parametric coefficients:
##              Estimate Std. Error z value Pr(>|z|)
## (Intercept) -2.617667   0.393674  -6.649 2.94e-11 ***
## instab      -0.120379   0.259801  -0.463 0.643113
## oil          1.074246   0.470396   2.284 0.022389 *
## cwar        -0.598469   0.320969  -1.865 0.062242 .
## lpop         0.116009   0.045152   2.569 0.010191 *
## lmnt         0.111640   0.043090   2.591 0.009573 **
## ethfrac      0.085478   0.196877   0.434 0.664165
## poldem       0.010101   0.008683   1.163 0.244704
## gdp         -0.211755   0.057078  -3.710 0.000207 ***
## relfrac      0.193637   0.257584   0.752 0.452206
## ---
## Signif. codes:  0 '***' 0.001 '**' 0.01 '*' 0.05 '.' 0.1 ' ' 1
##
##
## EQUATION 2
## Link function for mu2: probit
## Formula: onset ~ instab + oil + cwar + ncontig + nwstate + gdp
##
## Parametric coefficients:
##              Estimate Std. Error z value Pr(>|z|)
## (Intercept)  -0.8164     0.3808   -2.144    0.032 *
## instab        0.8721     0.6107    1.428    0.153
## oil          -0.9638     0.6069   -1.588    0.112
## cwar          0.2113     0.6875    0.307    0.759
## ncontig       0.5862     0.4968    1.180    0.238
## nwstate       2.6507     2.6735    0.991    0.321
## gdp           0.1058     0.1605    0.659    0.510
## ---
## Signif. codes:  0 '***' 0.001 '**' 0.01 '*' 0.05 '.' 0.1 ' ' 1
##
##
## n = 6326  total edf = 17
summary(pb)

##
## Family: binomial
## Link function: probit
##
## Formula:
## onset ~ instab + oil + cwar + ncontig + nwstate + lpop + lmnt +
##     ethfrac + poldem + gdp + relfrac
##
## Parametric coefficients:
##              Estimate Std. Error z value Pr(>|z|)
## (Intercept) -3.195155   0.305005 -10.476  < 2e-16 ***
```

```
## instab        0.261447   0.100910    2.591 0.009573 **
## oil           0.363115   0.122067    2.975 0.002933 **
## cwar         -0.378156   0.129964   -2.910 0.003618 **
## ncontig       0.155751   0.121656    1.280 0.200453
## nwstate       0.759499   0.163264    4.652 3.29e-06 ***
## lpop          0.104802   0.031235    3.355 0.000793 ***
## lmnt          0.091518   0.034332    2.666 0.007684 **
## ethfrac       0.078610   0.157388    0.499 0.617453
## poldem        0.009303   0.007004    1.328 0.184108
## gdp          -0.135517   0.028370   -4.777 1.78e-06 ***
## relfrac       0.127541   0.210798    0.605 0.545155
## ---
## Signif. codes:  0 '***' 0.001 '**' 0.01 '*' 0.05 '.' 0.1 ' ' 1
##
##
## R-sq.(adj) =  0.0314   Deviance explained = 10.5%
## UBRE = -0.845  Scale est. = 1          n = 6326
```

Many predictors influence the onset of civil war, but the pb model does not shed light on the political mechanisms involving both oppositions and governments, which are captured by bpo0 instead. For example, in the pb model, gdp shows a negative and statistically significant effect on the likelihood of civil war onset. This may imply that states with greater economic capacity are either more effective at deterring insurgents or that potential rebels are less inclined to challenge governments due to higher opportunity costs or perhaps a combination of these elements. Conversely, in bpo0, gdp retains a negative and statistically significant effect in the rebel equation (suggesting that as gdp increases, potential rebel groups are less likely to engage governments), but shows no significant impact in the government equation.

The probabilities for all possible outcomes are shown below.

```
nd <- data.frame(t(apply(war, 2, FUN = median)))

copula.prob(bpo0, y1 = 1, y2 = 1, newdata = nd, intervals = TRUE)
```

```
##          p12         2.5%         97.5%
##   0.01318276 0.007434751 0.01691572
```

```
predict(pb, nd, type = "response")
```

```
##           1
## 0.01195086
```

```
copula.prob(bpo0, y1 = 1, y2 = 0, newdata = nd, intervals = TRUE)
```

```
##          p12         2.5%         97.5%
##   0.03510232 0.006345774 0.09409629
```

```
copula.prob(bpo0, y1 = 0, y2 = 1, newdata = nd, intervals = TRUE)
```

```
##          p12         2.5%         97.5%
##   0.2598366 0.04845854 0.5060103
```

```
copula.prob(bpo0, y1 = 0, y2 = 0, newdata = nd, intervals = TRUE)
```

```
##          p12         2.5%         97.5%
##   0.6918783 0.3853666 0.8277869
```

Given that $\theta = 0$ in `bpo0`, the results for the probability of civil war are very similar in both `bpo0` and `pb` models, at 1.3% and 1.2%, respectively. That is, for typical values of the covariates in both the rebel and government equations, such low probabilities indicate that simultaneous action from both decision makers is relatively rare. However, the partial observability model provides additional insights. Specifically, the probability of a challenge occurring without a government response is 3.5%. In contrast, the probability of a forceful response arising without an initial challenge is 26%, suggesting a proactive stance against potential threats. Furthermore, there is a high probability (69.2%) that neither side engages in confrontation, indicating a prevailing environment of stability. These findings emphasize the complex interaction between economic variables and political decision-making, highlighting the value of capturing such nuanced dynamics.

Part III

Mixed Types of Marginals

8

Ordinal and continuous outcomes

This chapter delves into the joint regression modeling of ordinal and continuous responses, using the method proposed by Hohberg et al. [2021]. The focus is on a case study examining the relationship between happiness (an ordinal response) and economic prosperity (a continuous outcome) across countries, conditional on health and social variables. Mixed outcomes of this nature have been studied in various fields such as economics [Spiess, 2006, Teimourian et al., 2015] and medicine [Ivanova et al., 2016, Delporte et al., 2024].

The framework explored here captures the dependence between well-being and economic performance, while taking into account diverse influences such as social support, health outcomes and freedom. The approach not only enables the simultaneous analysis of these multifaceted outcomes but also sheds light on shared and distinct drivers of happiness and prosperity, offering deeper insights into how these elements collectively shape societal wellness.

8.1 Happiness and economic prosperity

The data are sourced from the 2019 World Happiness Report, an annual publication of the United Nations Sustainable Development Solutions Network [Helliwell et al., 2019]. The aim is to simultaneously model happiness and economic performance [Oswald, 1997], conditional on covariate information. The outcomes are subjective well-being `score` (ranging from 1 for low to 4 for high happiness) and `gdp` (gross domestic product per capita). The set of covariates consists of healthy life expectancy (`hle`), social support (`support`), freedom to make life choices (`freedom`), generosity (`generosity`) and perception of corruption (`corruption`). The dataset contains 155 observations.

Happiness and economic performance are closely interrelated. Economic prosperity often enhances quality of life, potentially increasing happiness among citizens. Conversely, higher levels of happiness can foster social cohesion and improve productivity, which in turn benefits economic outcomes. Joint modeling captures this interdependence, offering a more nuanced understanding of the problem and thus providing policymakers with insights to develop more comprehensive strategies that integrate economic goals with well-being factors.

8.2 Model

Consider a pair of ordinal and continuous variables (Y_1, Y_2). The ordinal variable Y_1 is defined as

$$Y_1 = \begin{cases} 1 & \text{if} \quad Y_1^* \le c_1 \\ 2 & \text{if} \quad c_1 < Y_1^* \le c_2 \\ \;\;\vdots \\ k & \text{if} \quad c_{k-1} < Y_1^* \le c_k \\ \;\;\vdots \\ K & \text{if} \quad c_{K-1} < Y_1^* \le c_K \end{cases},$$

where $Y_1^* \sim D_1(\mu_1, \sigma_1)$ and $D_1(\cdot, \cdot)$ is either a Gaussian or logistic distribution with $g_{\mu_1}(\mu_1) = \eta_{\mu_1}(\boldsymbol{x}_{\mu_1}; \boldsymbol{\beta}_{\mu_1})$ and $\sigma_1 = 1$. The unknown cutoff points $c_1, c_2, \ldots, c_{K-1}$ are real numbers that satisfy the monotonic condition $-\infty = c_0 < c_1 < c_2 < \cdots < c_{K-1} < c_K = \infty$. The continuous outcome is modeled as $Y_2 \sim D_2(\mu_2, \sigma_2)$, where $g_{\mu_2}(\mu_2) = \eta_{\mu_2}(\boldsymbol{x}_{\mu_2}; \boldsymbol{\beta}_{\mu_2})$ and $g_{\sigma_2}(\sigma_2) = \eta_{\sigma_2}(\boldsymbol{x}_{\sigma_2}; \boldsymbol{\beta}_{\sigma_2})$, using any of the two parameter distributions reported in Table 1.3. The extension to three parameters will be addressed in future work.

Using a copula function $C(\cdot, \cdot; \theta)$, where $g_\theta(\theta) = \eta_\theta(\boldsymbol{x}_\theta; \boldsymbol{\beta}_\theta)$, the joint CDF can be written as

$$\mathbb{P}(Y_1 \le k, Y_2 \le y_2) = C(F_1(c_k - \mu_1), F_2(y_2; \mu_2, \sigma_2); \theta),$$

where $F_1(c_k - \mu_1)$ denotes the CDF of either a standard Gaussian or standard logistic distribution and $F_2(y_2; \mu_2, \sigma_2)$ is the CDF associated with the continuous response. The joint PDF, $f_{12}(k, y_2; c_k, c_{k-1}, \mu_1, \mu_2, \sigma_2, \theta)$, is

$$\begin{cases} \dfrac{\partial C(F_1(c_k - \mu_1), F_2(y_2; \mu_2, \sigma_2); \theta)}{\partial F_2(y_2; \mu_2, \sigma_2)} f_2(y_2; \mu_2, \sigma_2) & \text{for } k = 1 \\ \left(\dfrac{\partial C(F_1(c_k - \mu_1), F_2(y_2; \mu_2, \sigma_2); \theta)}{\partial F_2(y_2; \mu_2, \sigma_2)} - \dfrac{\partial C(F_1(c_{k-1} - \mu_1), F_2(y_2; \mu_2, \sigma_2); \theta)}{\partial F_2(y_2; \mu_2, \sigma_2)} \right) f_2(y_2; \mu_2, \sigma_2) & \text{for } 1 < k \le K \end{cases},$$

$$(8.1)$$

where $f_2(y_2; \mu_2, \sigma_2)$ is the PDF of Y_2.

8.3   Log-likelihood

Using equation (8.1), for a random sample $(y_{i1}, y_{i2}, \boldsymbol{x}_i)_{i=1}^n$, where the covariate vector $\boldsymbol{x}_i$ is the union of $\boldsymbol{x}_{i\mu_1}, \boldsymbol{x}_{i\mu_2}, \boldsymbol{x}_{i\sigma_2}$ and $\boldsymbol{x}_{i\theta}$, the log-likelihood of the mixed ordinal and continuous outcomes copula regression model is

$$\ell(\boldsymbol{\beta}) = \sum_{i=1}^n \left[\sum_{k=1}^K \mathbb{1}_{y_{i1}=k} \log \left\{ \frac{\partial C(F_1(c_k - \mu_{i1}), F_2(y_{i2}; \mu_{i2}, \sigma_{i2}); \theta_i)}{\partial F_2(y_{i2}; \mu_{i2}, \sigma_{i2})} \right. \right.$$
$$\left. \left. - \frac{\partial C(F_1(c_{k-1} - \mu_{i1}), F_2(y_{i2}; \mu_{i2}, \sigma_{i2}); \theta_i)}{\partial F_2(y_{i2}; \mu_{i2}, \sigma_{i2})} \right\} + \log \left\{ f_2(y_{i2}; \mu_{i2}, \sigma_{i2}) \right\} \right],$$

where $\boldsymbol{\beta} = (\boldsymbol{c}^\top, \boldsymbol{\beta}_{\mu_1}^\top, \boldsymbol{\beta}_{\mu_2}^\top, \boldsymbol{\beta}_{\sigma_2}^\top, \boldsymbol{\beta}_\theta^\top)^\top$, with $\boldsymbol{c}$ including all the cutoff parameters, is the overall model coefficient vector. Note that when $k = 1$,

$$\frac{\partial C(F_1(c_{k-1} - \mu_{i1}), F_2(y_{i2}; \mu_{i2}, \sigma_{i2}); \theta_i)}{\partial F_2(y_{i2}; \mu_{i2}, \sigma_{i2})} = 0.$$

8.4 Model fitting

Several models based on different combinations of copulae and marginal distributions were evaluated. Given the small sample size, smooth effects were not considered. Based on convergence and residual checks, as well as parsimony and information-based criteria, the adopted model is

```
library(GJRM); library(GJRM.data)
data(happy)

eq1 <- score  ~ support + hle + freedom + generosity + corruption
eq2 <- gdp    ~ support + hle + freedom + generosity + corruption
eq3 <-        ~ support + hle + freedom + generosity + corruption

out <- gjrm(list(eq1, eq2, eq3, ~ 1), data = happy,
        margins = c("ord.probit", "LO"), copula = "AMH", model = "B")
```

where all the distributional parameters but θ are specified as functions of covariate effects.

```
conv.check(out)
```

```
##
## Maximum absolute gradient value: 9.442575e-09
## Observed information matrix is positive definite
```

```
res.check(out, intervals = TRUE)
```

Convergence checks are satisfactory, and the residual plot shown in Figure 8.1 supports the selected marginal distribution for the continuous outcome.

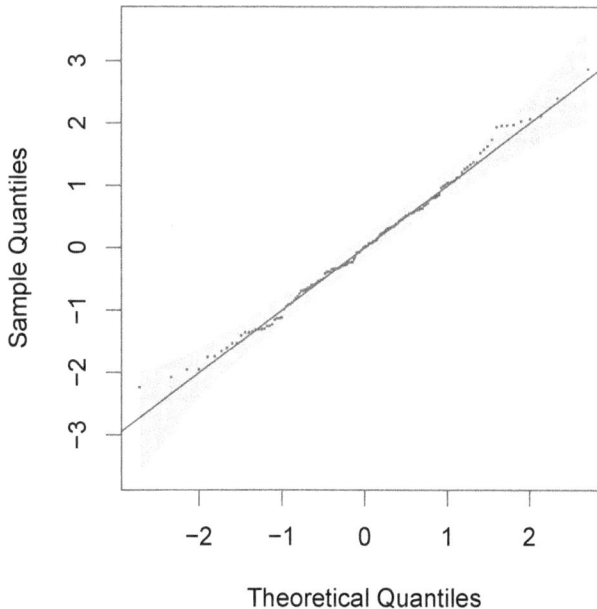

FIGURE 8.1 Normal Q–Q plot of normalized quantile residuals for the continuous outcome, derived from an AMH copula model with ord.probit and LO margins fitted to the happy data.

The findings are summarized as follows.

```
summary(out)
```

```
##
## COPULA: AMH
## MARGIN 1: Ordinal
## MARGIN 2: Logistic
##
## EQUATION 1
## Link function for mu1: probit
## Formula: score ~ support + hle + freedom + generosity + corruption
##
## Parametric coefficients:
##             Estimate Std. Error z value Pr(>|z|)
## support       2.9443     0.5590   5.267 1.39e-07 ***
## hle           3.7509     0.6636   5.653 1.58e-08 ***
## freedom       3.2539     0.9160   3.552 0.000382 ***
## generosity    0.5920     1.1390   0.520 0.603235
## corruption   -1.0004     1.4103  -0.709 0.478103
## ---
## Signif. codes:  0 '***' 0.001 '**' 0.01 '*' 0.05 '.' 0.1 ' ' 1
##
##
## EQUATION 2
## Link function for mu2: identity
## Formula: gdp ~ support + hle + freedom + generosity + corruption
##
## Parametric coefficients:
##             Estimate Std. Error z value Pr(>|z|)
## (Intercept) -0.30048    0.06713  -4.476 7.61e-06 ***
## support      0.30222    0.06919   4.368 1.25e-05 ***
## hle          1.13576    0.08417  13.494  < 2e-16 ***
## freedom     -0.04900    0.09302  -0.527 0.598313
## generosity  -0.09457    0.13742  -0.688 0.491351
## corruption   0.40901    0.12422   3.293 0.000992 ***
## ---
## Signif. codes:  0 '***' 0.001 '**' 0.01 '*' 0.05 '.' 0.1 ' ' 1
##
##
## EQUATION 3
## Link function for sigma2: log
## Formula: ~support + hle + freedom + generosity + corruption
##
## Parametric coefficients:
##             Estimate Std. Error z value Pr(>|z|)
## (Intercept) -1.6290     0.3529  -4.617 3.90e-06 ***
## support      0.2358     0.3776   0.624  0.53232
## hle         -2.2362     0.4923  -4.542 5.57e-06 ***
## freedom      1.7901     0.6120   2.925  0.00345 **
## generosity  -0.0134     0.8881  -0.015  0.98796
```

```
## corruption    -0.5530      0.9217  -0.600  0.54853
## ---
## Signif. codes:  0 '***' 0.001 '**' 0.01 '*' 0.05 '.' 0.1 ' ' 1
##
##
## EQUATION 4
## Link function for theta: atanh
## Formula: ~1
##
## Parametric coefficients:
##              Estimate Std. Error z value Pr(>|z|)
## (Intercept)    1.1348     0.3235   3.508 0.000452 ***
## ---
## Signif. codes:  0 '***' 0.001 '**' 0.01 '*' 0.05 '.' 0.1 ' ' 1
##
##
## sigma2 = 0.109(0.0791,0.155)
## theta = 0.813(0.541,0.935)
## n = 155   total edf = 21
```

The estimated copula parameter is positive and significant, suggesting that, after controlling for covariates, unmeasured variables, such as cultural values and social norms, influence both subjective well-being and economic outcomes.

The results from the first equation indicate that **support**, **hle** and **freedom** significantly increase the likelihood of experiencing a high level of happiness, highlighting the value of social support networks, health and personal liberties in enhancing quality of life. In contrast, **generosity** and **corruption** do not appear to influence the response, possibly due to the small sample size, although the estimated effects align with expectations.

In the second equation, **support**, **hle** and **corruption** show positive and significant impacts on economic performance, emphasizing the relevance of social support systems and health indicators in driving economic growth. The positive effect of corruption warrants further investigation to fully understand the underlying mechanisms and conditions leading to such a finding. The results also indicate that the variability of **gdp** is influenced by **hle** and **freedom**; higher **hle** is associated with reduced **gdp** variability, likely due to a healthier, more stable workforce, while greater **freedom** increases variability, suggesting that although it fosters growth, it may also introduce economic uncertainty.

The expectation of a continuous response conditional on an ordinal outcome is defined as

$$\mathbb{E}(Y_2|Y_1 = k) = \frac{1}{F_1(c_k - \mu_1) - F_1(c_{k-1} - \mu_1)} \int y_2 f_{12}(k, y_2; c_k, c_{k-1}, \mu_1, \mu_2, \sigma_2, \theta) dy_2,$$

where the integration is over the support of y_2 and $F_1(c_{k-1} - \mu_1) = 0$ when $k = 1$. Intervals are conveniently obtained through posterior simulation.

For a typical country, the conditional means of `gdp` across the four levels of happiness are displayed in Figure 8.2.

```
nd <- data.frame(support = 1.27, hle = 0.79, freedom = 0.42,
                 generosity = 0.18, corruption = 0.08)
m <- l <- u <- NA

for(i in 1:4) {
  res   <- cond.mv(out, eq = 2, y1 = i, newdata = nd)
  l[i] <- res$res[1]; m[i] <- res$res[2]; u[i] <- res$res[3]
}

plot(m, ylim = range(c(l, u)), xlab = "Subjective well-being",
     ylab = "Conditional mean", pch = 16, xaxt = "n")
axis(1, at = 1:4, labels = c("low", "medium-low", "medium", "high"))

for(i in 1:4) arrows(i, l[i], i, u[i], angle = 90, code = 3, length = 0.1)
```

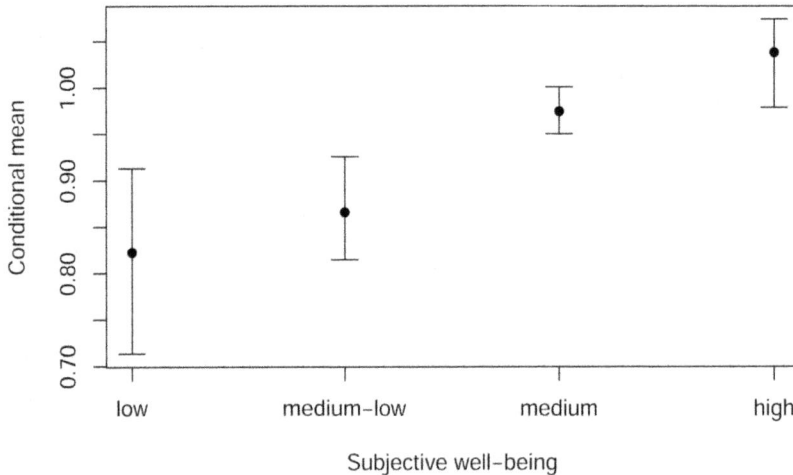

FIGURE 8.2 Conditional means and 95% intervals of gross domestic product per capita across subjective well-being categories for a typical country, derived from an `AMH` copula model with `ord.probit` and `LO` margins fitted to the `happy` data.

The plot reveals an upward trend, with economic performance improving as happiness increases. For example, the expected `gdp` is 0.82 at the lowest happiness level and rises to 1.04 at the highest, suggesting that happier societies tend to experience stronger economic outcomes.

The probability of achieving a given happiness level, conditional on a specific value of `gdp`, can also be of interest and is obtained by dividing equation (8.1) by $f_2(y_2; \mu_2, \sigma_2)$.

```
gdp.v <- c(0.5, 1, 1.5)
for(i in 1:3) print(round(copula.prob(out, y1 = 4, y2 = gdp.v[i],
                          newdata = nd, cond = 2, intervals = TRUE), 2))
```

```
##    p12 2.5% 97.5%
##   0.06 0.02  0.16
##   0.29 0.19  0.39
##   0.42 0.28  0.54
```

With a gdp of 0.5, the probability of high happiness is only 0.06, but it increases to 0.42 at a gdp of 1.5. This indicates that stronger economic performance, likely through better living standards and access to resources, contributes significantly to well-being. However, the widening confidence intervals at higher gdp levels suggest that other factors may also play a role in this relationship.

9

Binary and continuous outcomes

Studies often involve bivariate binary and continuous responses. In healthcare utilization, for example, researchers may be interested in quantifying the impact of managed care interventions on healthcare costs and mortality rates [McCulloch, 2008], and in investigating the relationship between hospitalization costs and the use of intensive care units [de Oliveira et al., 2019]. Toxicity research also provides relevant instances, such as analyses exploring the effects of toxic agents on fetal weight and malformation status [Fitzmaurice and Laird, 1995, Najita et al., 2009].

In this chapter, the copula regression model by Klein et al. [2019] is employed to examine how various individual characteristics influence HIV status and CD4 counts, while accounting for their dependence. Predictive analyses are also performed to evaluate the outcomes across different scenarios.

9.1 HIV status and CD4 counts

The study utilizes fictitious data designed to closely mirror the characteristics and patterns observed in the Africa Centre Demographic Information System for women [Tanser et al., 2007]. The dataset includes information on 2,645 subjects, covering HIV status (`hiv`), CD4 count measurements (`cd4.count`), `age`, `location`, `marital` status, presence of household `water`, `education` and distances to the nearest primary and secondary schools (`distance1` and `distance2`, respectively).

Simultaneously modeling HIV status and CD4 counts provides a more comprehensive understanding of their mutual influence and the impact of shared risk factors. This approach yields deeper insights into the relationships between the responses and covariates, enabling thorough predictions and supporting the development of targeted public health interventions to improve HIV prevention and CD4 count management.

9.2 Model

Let us assume that Y_1 is a binary response that follows a Bernoulli distribution, $Y_1 \sim \text{Ber}(\mu_1)$, where $g_{\mu_1}(\mu_1) = \eta_{\mu_1}(\boldsymbol{x}_{\mu_1}; \boldsymbol{\beta}_{\mu_1})$. Let also Y_2 be a continuous outcome specified as $Y_2 \sim D_2(\mu_2, \sigma_2, \nu_2)$, where $D_2(\cdot, \cdot, \cdot)$ is represented using any of the distributions listed in Table 1.3, $g_{\mu_2}(\mu_2) = \eta_{\mu_2}(\boldsymbol{x}_{\mu_2}; \boldsymbol{\beta}_{\mu_2})$, $g_{\sigma_2}(\sigma_2) = \eta_{\sigma_2}(\boldsymbol{x}_{\sigma_2}; \boldsymbol{\beta}_{\sigma_2})$ and $g_{\nu_2}(\nu_2) = \eta_{\nu_2}(\boldsymbol{x}_{\nu_2}; \boldsymbol{\beta}_{\mu_2})$. Note that, although `cd4.count` is a discrete variable, the best fit was produced by a continuous distribution, likely due to the wide range of CD4 values.

DOI: 10.1201/9781003593195-9

Define $F_1(y_1; \mu_1)$ and $F_2(y_2; \mu_2, \sigma_2, \nu_2)$ as the CDFs of Y_1 and Y_2, respectively. Using a copula function $C(\cdot, \cdot; \theta)$, where $g_\theta(\theta) = \eta_\theta(\boldsymbol{x}_\theta; \boldsymbol{\beta}_\theta)$, the joint probabilities associated with the pair (Y_1, Y_2) can be expressed as

$$\mathbb{P}(Y_1 = 0, Y_2 \leq y_2) = C(F_1(0; \mu_1), F_2(y_2; \mu_2, \sigma_2, \nu_2); \theta)$$

and

$$\mathbb{P}(Y_1 = 1, Y_2 \leq y_2) = F_2(y_2; \mu_2, \sigma_2, \nu_2) - C(F_1(0; \mu_1), F_2(y_2; \mu_2, \sigma_2, \nu_2); \theta).$$

The resulting mixed binary-continuous density is

$$
\begin{aligned}
f_{12}(y_1, y_2; \mu_1, \mu_2, \sigma_2, \nu_2, \theta) = & \left\{ \frac{\partial C(F_1(0; \mu_1), F_2(y_2; \mu_2, \sigma_2, \nu_2); \theta)}{\partial F_2(y_2; \mu_2, \sigma_2, \nu_2)} \right\}^{1-y_1} \\
& \times \left\{ 1 - \frac{\partial C(F_1(0; \mu_1), F_2(y_2; \mu_2, \sigma_2, \nu_2); \theta)}{\partial F_2(y_2; \mu_2, \sigma_2, \nu_2)} \right\}^{y_1}, \\
& \times f_2(y_2; \mu_2, \sigma_2, \nu_2)
\end{aligned}
\tag{9.1}
$$

where $f_2(y_2; \mu_2, \sigma_2, \nu_2) = \frac{\partial F_2(y_2; \mu_2, \sigma_2, \nu_2)}{\partial y_2}$ is the marginal PDF of Y_2.

9.3 Log-likelihood

Using equation (9.1), for a random sample $(y_{i1}, y_{i2}, \boldsymbol{x}_i)_{i=1}^n$, where the covariate vector $\boldsymbol{x}_i$ is the union of $\boldsymbol{x}_{i\mu_1}$, $\boldsymbol{x}_{i\mu_2}$, $\boldsymbol{x}_{i\sigma_2}$, $\boldsymbol{x}_{i\nu_2}$ and $\boldsymbol{x}_{i\theta}$, the log-likelihood function of the mixed binary-continuous outcomes copula regression model is

$$
\begin{aligned}
\ell(\boldsymbol{\beta}) = \sum_{i=1}^n & \left[(1 - y_{i1}) \log \left\{ F_{1|2}(0|y_{i2}; \mu_{i1}, \mu_{i2}, \sigma_{i2}, \nu_{i2}, \theta_i) \right\} \right. \\
& \left. + y_{i1} \log \left\{ 1 - F_{1|2}(0|y_{i2}; \mu_{i1}, \mu_{i2}, \sigma_{i2}, \nu_{i2}, \theta_i) \right\} + \log \left\{ f_2(y_{i2}; \mu_{i2}, \sigma_{i2}, \nu_{i2}) \right\} \right]
\end{aligned}
,
$$

where

$$
F_{1|2}(0|y_{i2}; \mu_{i1}, \mu_{i2}, \sigma_{i2}, \nu_{i2}, \theta_i) = \frac{\partial C\left(F_1(0; \mu_{i1}), F_2(y_{i2}; \mu_{i2}, \sigma_{i2}, \nu_{i2}); \theta_i\right)}{\partial F_2(y_{i2}; \mu_{i2}, \sigma_{i2}, \nu_{i2})}
\tag{9.2}
$$

is the conditional CDF of $Y_1 = 0$ given y_2, and $\boldsymbol{\beta} = (\boldsymbol{\beta}_{\mu_1}^\top, \boldsymbol{\beta}_{\mu_2}^\top, \boldsymbol{\beta}_{\sigma_2}^\top, \boldsymbol{\beta}_{\nu_2}^\top, \boldsymbol{\beta}_\theta^\top)^\top$ is the overall regression coefficient vector.

9.4 Model fitting

The two main equations, for μ_1 and μ_2, are specified as

```
library(GJRM); library(GJRM.data)
data(cd4)

eq1 <- hiv        ~ s(age) + distance1 + distance2 + marital + water +
                    education
eq2 <- cd4.count  ~ s(age) + distance1 + distance2 + marital + water +
                    education
```

Parameters σ_2, ν_2 and θ can also be defined as functions of additive predictors using the generic formula

```
eqg <-        ~ s(age) + distance1 + distance2 + marital +
              water + education
```

The link function for $g_{\mu_1}(\cdot)$ was chosen by fitting three binary models using `mgcv::gam()`, based on the `logit`, `cloglog` and `probit` links, respectively. The `logit` was most supported by information-based criteria, although the specific choice of link function did not affect the substantive conclusions. For `cd4.count`, the best fit was produced by the Dagum distribution with μ_2 specified as a function of an additive predictor, and σ_2 and ν_2 estimated without accounting for covariate effects. Several copulae were evaluated, including the case where θ was modeled using `eqg`. The preferred model was the 270° rotated Gumbel copula, with the dependence parameter estimated without taking into account covariate effects.

```
out <- gjrm(list(eq1, eq2), data = cd4, margins = c("logit", "DAGUM"),
            copula = "G270", model = "B")
conv.check(out)

##
## Maximum absolute gradient value: 5.929902e-12
## Observed information matrix is positive definite

res.check(out, intervals = TRUE)
```

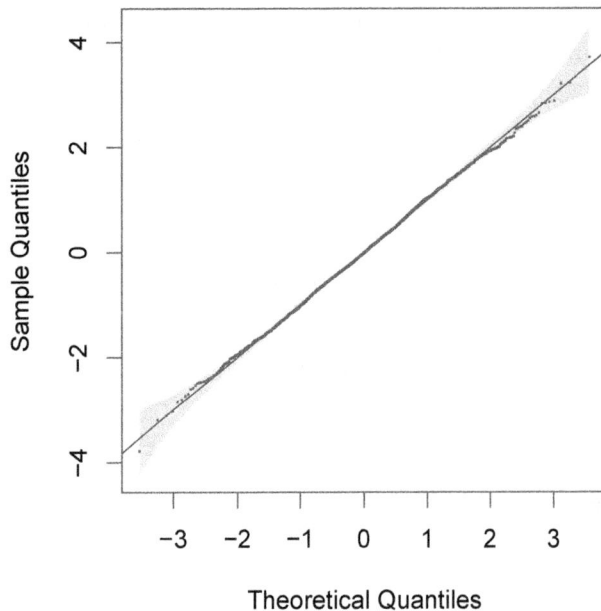

FIGURE 9.1 Normal Q–Q plot of normalized quantile residuals, derived from a 270° Gumbel copula additive distributional regression model with `logit` and `DAGUM` margins fitted to the `cd4` data.

Convergence checks and the residual plot reported in Figure 9.1 are satisfactory.

The findings from the fitted model are summarized in the following outputs and commentary.

`summary(out)`

```
##
## COPULA: 270° Gumbel
## MARGIN 1: Bernoulli
## MARGIN 2: Dagum
##
## EQUATION 1
## Link function for mu1: logit
## Formula: hiv ~ s(age) + distance1 + distance2 + marital + water +
## education
## Parametric coefficients:
##                          Estimate Std. Error z value Pr(>|z|)
## (Intercept)              -1.33339    0.22669  -5.882 4.06e-09 ***
## distance1                -0.12233    0.06786  -1.803  0.07142 .
## distance2                -0.02096    0.03762  -0.557  0.57742
## maritalEngaged           -0.10357    0.29781  -0.348  0.72802
## maritalMarried           -0.57256    0.18989  -3.015  0.00257 **
## maritalNever Married      0.33443    0.17111   1.954  0.05064 .
## maritalPolygamous        -0.41866    0.32182  -1.301  0.19329
## maritalUnder Legal Age    0.37966    0.25786   1.472  0.14092
## water                     0.31509    0.11544   2.730  0.00634 **
## educationNone             0.01445    0.17209   0.084  0.93310
## educationPrimary          0.27627    0.15162   1.822  0.06843 .
## educationUpper Secondary  0.03755    0.11511   0.326  0.74424
## ---
## Signif. codes:  0 '***' 0.001 '**' 0.01 '*' 0.05 '.' 0.1 ' ' 1
##
## Approximate significance of smooth terms:
##          edf Ref.df Chi.sq p-value
## s(age) 5.903  6.915  193.2  <2e-16 ***
## ---
## Signif. codes:  0 '***' 0.001 '**' 0.01 '*' 0.05 '.' 0.1 ' ' 1
##
##
## EQUATION 2
## Link function for mu2: log
## Formula: cd4.count ~ s(age) + distance1 + distance2 + marital + water +
##     education
##
## Parametric coefficients:
##                      Estimate Std. Error z value Pr(>|z|)
## (Intercept)          6.867278   0.046016 149.238   <2e-16 ***
## distance1            0.030516   0.012996   2.348   0.0189 *
## distance2           -0.012499   0.007314  -1.709   0.0875 .
## maritalEngaged       0.014420   0.065125   0.221   0.8248
## maritalMarried       0.065509   0.035807   1.830   0.0673 .
## maritalNever Married -0.047578   0.033544  -1.418   0.1561
## maritalPolygamous    0.024017   0.059206   0.406   0.6850
```

```
## maritalUnder Legal Age    -0.028130   0.049664  -0.566   0.5711
## water                       0.019133   0.022303   0.858   0.3910
## educationNone               0.040193   0.032879   1.222   0.2215
## educationPrimary            0.008642   0.030643   0.282   0.7779
## educationUpper Secondary   -0.004128   0.023778  -0.174   0.8622
## ---
## Signif. codes:  0 '***' 0.001 '**' 0.01 '*' 0.05 '.' 0.1 ' ' 1
##
## Approximate significance of smooth terms:
##           edf Ref.df Chi.sq p-value
## s(age) 5.934  7.085  71.34  <2e-16 ***
## ---
## Signif. codes:  0 '***' 0.001 '**' 0.01 '*' 0.05 '.' 0.1 ' ' 1
##
##
## sigma2 = 6.05(5.7,6.6)  nu2 = 0.338(0.309,0.371)
## theta = -2.3(-2.44,-2.15)
## n = 2645   total edf = 38.8
```

Married women have 43.6% lower odds of being HIV positive compared to previously married women. This trend is often attributed to the stability of monogamous relationships, which is also associated with improved CD4 counts. Conversely, women who have never been married exhibit 39.7% higher odds of being HIV positive compared to formerly married women, which aligns with the assumption that never-married individuals might engage in more transient relationships or have several sexual partners. Other marital statuses, such as engaged or polygamous, do not show significant effects on either HIV risk or CD4 counts, which is somewhat unexpected. For instance, polygamous relationships are generally associated with higher HIV vulnerability. The lack of statistical significance might stem from the limited representation of these subgroups in this dataset.

The relationships between distance to primary schools and the two outcomes suggest that women living farther from schools may have higher CD4 counts and a lower probability of being HIV positive. This finding may reflect underlying socio-environmental variables, such as differences in healthcare access, population density and local health infrastructure, which vary with distance to schools and may indirectly influence both HIV prevalence and immune health outcomes. The positive relation between water availability and HIV status contradicts typical preconceptions because improved access to clean water is generally associated with lower health risks. However, in some contexts, areas with better infrastructure may also be more urbanized, which often corresponds to higher HIV rates. Although education is often one of the key covariates for many health outcomes, it does not appear to play an important role in this analysis.

```
par(mfrow = c(1, 2))
plot(out, eq = 1); plot(out, eq = 2)
```

The nonlinear effects of age, displayed in Figure 9.2, show that the propensity of being HIV positive increases until approximately age 35 before declining, while CD4 counts follow the opposite pattern, decreasing until 35 and then rising. These trends likely reflect a complex interplay of behavioral and social factors, such as riskier sexual practices and delayed healthcare access during early adulthood, which contribute to both higher HIV risk and lower CD4 counts. As individuals age, they may adopt healthier behaviors, access better healthcare and adhere more to treatment, leading to lower HIV rates and improved immune function.

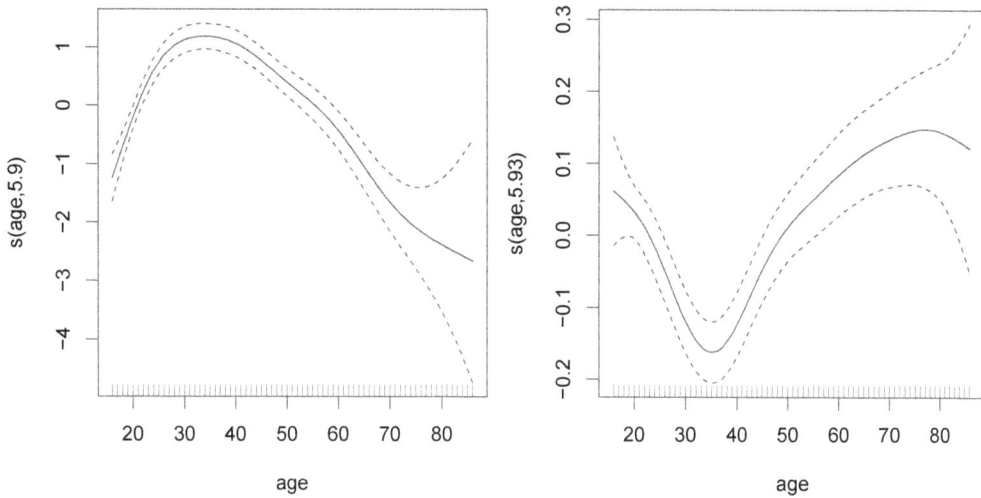

FIGURE 9.2 Estimated smooth effects (with associated 95% intervals) of `age` on the scales of the additive predictors of μ_1 and μ_2, derived from a 270° rotated Gumbel copula additive distributional regression model with `logit` and `DAGUM` margins fitted to the `cd4` data.

The copula parameter hints at a negative association between HIV status and CD4 counts. The 270° rotation of the Gumbel copula is typically used to capture left-tail dependence. In this case, lower CD4 counts are linked to a higher probability of being HIV positive, which is consistent with the biological mechanism of HIV infection.

Figure 9.3 reports $\mathbb{P}(\texttt{hiv} = 1 | \texttt{cd4.count})$, derived as one minus equation (9.2), for a typical woman across a grid of `cd4.count` values.

```
nd <- data.frame(age = 33, location = "RUR", distance1 = 1.150,
                 distance2 = 1.850, marital = "Never Married",
                 water = 1, education = "Upper Secondary")

lg <- 25; cd4g <- seq(400, 1000, length.out = lg)
res <- data.frame(matrix(nrow = lg, ncol = 3))

for(i in 1:lg) res[i, ] <- copula.prob(out, y1 = 1, y2 = cd4g[i], cond = 2,
                   newdata = nd, intervals = TRUE,  n.sim = 1000)

plot(cd4g, res[, 1], type = "l", ylab = "P(hiv = 1|cd4)",
     xlab = "cd4", ylim = range(res))
lines(cd4g, res[, 2], lty = 2); lines(cd4g, res[, 3], lty = 2)
```

For a CD4 count around 400 cells/mm^3, the probability of being HIV positive is high, indicating greater immune vulnerability. As CD4 counts increase, the probability of HIV positivity declines. Notably, when CD4 counts range between 600 and 700, the probability of being HIV positive is roughly half that observed when CD4 counts are around 400, emphasizing the need to monitor CD4 levels for managing HIV progression and maintaining immune health.

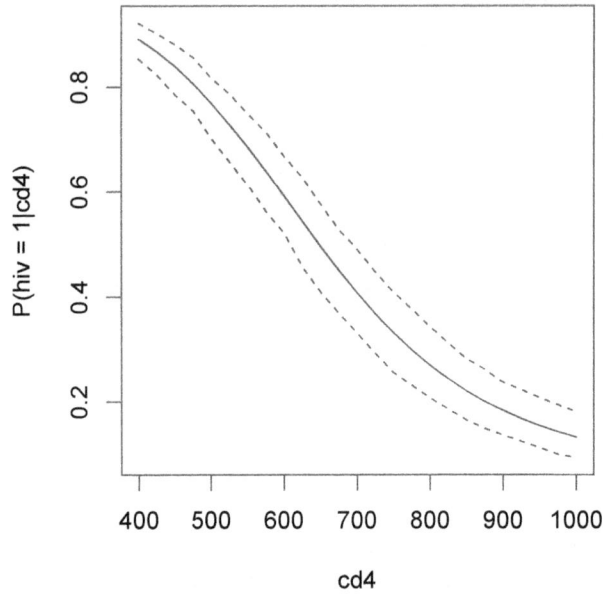

FIGURE 9.3 Conditional probabilities and their associated 95% intervals for `hiv` $= 1$ given `cd4.count` for a typical woman, derived from a 270° rotated Gumbel copula additive distributional regression model with `logit` and `DAGUM` margins fitted to the `cd4` data.

The conditional expectations of the continuous response are defined as

$$\mathbb{E}(Y_2|Y_1 = 0) = \frac{1}{F_1(0;\mu_1)} \int y_2 F_{1|2}(0|y_2;\mu_1,\mu_2,\sigma_2,\nu_2,\theta) f_2(y_2;\mu_2,\sigma_2,\nu_2) dy_2$$

and

$$\mathbb{E}(Y_2|Y_1 = 1) = \frac{1}{1 - F_1(0;\mu_1)} \int y_2 \{1 - F_{1|2}(0|y_2;\mu_1,\mu_2,\sigma_2,\nu_2,\theta)\} f_2(y_2;\mu_2,\sigma_2,\nu_2) dy_2,$$

where, in each case, the integration is performed over the support of y_2, and intervals are conveniently obtained through posterior simulation.

```
cond.mv(out, eq = 2, y1 = 1, newdata = nd)
```

```
##
## Conditional mean with 95% interval:
##
## 468 (448,491)
```

```
cond.mv(out, eq = 2, y1 = 0, newdata = nd)
```

```
##
## Conditional mean with 95% interval:
##
## 802 (776,843)
```

The predicted mean for a typical HIV-positive woman is 468, with a narrow interval, which is below the normal range of 500–1500. This result suggests a potentially vulnerable immune system, highlighting the woman's increased susceptibility to opportunistic infections and the need for timely interventions, such as antiretroviral therapy. In contrast, the mean CD4 count for a typical HIV-negative woman is significantly higher, indicating healthier immune function. These findings highlight the critical role of early detection and treatment in preventing significant immune system deterioration.

9.5 A semicontinuous extension

GJRM supports the specification of copula models for mixed binary and semicontinuous outcomes using the Tweedie distribution discussed in Section 1.1.2. This approach is suitable for situations where Y_2 contains a significant proportion of zeros, along with a skewed distribution of positive values.

In this case, the joint density $f_{12}(y_1, y_2; \mu_1, \mu_2, \sigma_2, \nu_2, \theta)$ is built by considering the four possible combinations of values that (Y_1, Y_2) can take. Specifically,

$$
f_{12}(y_1, y_2; \mu_1, \mu_2, \sigma_2, \nu_2) =
$$

$$
\begin{cases}
C\left(F_1(0; \mu_1), F_2(0; \mu_2, \sigma_2, \nu_2); \theta\right) & \text{if } y_1 = 0 \text{ and } y_2 = 0 \\
F_2(0; \mu_2, \sigma_2, \nu_2) - C\left(F_1(0; \mu_1), F_2(0; \mu_2, \sigma_2, \nu_2); \theta\right) & \text{if } y_1 = 1 \text{ and } y_2 = 0 \\
f_2(y_2; \mu_2, \sigma_2, \nu_2) \frac{\partial C(F_1(0; \mu_1), F_2(y_2; \mu_2, \sigma_2, \nu_2); \theta)}{\partial F_2(y_2; \mu_2, \sigma_2, \nu_2)} & \text{if } y_1 = 0 \text{ and } y_2 > 0 \\
f_2(y_2; \mu_2, \sigma_2, \nu_2) \left\{1 - \frac{\partial C(F_1(0; \mu_1), F_2(y_2; \mu_2, \sigma_2, \nu_2); \theta)}{\partial F_2(y_2; \mu_2, \sigma_2, \nu_2)}\right\} & \text{if } y_1 = 1 \text{ and } y_2 > 0
\end{cases}
$$

where F_2 and f_2 denote the CDF and PDF of the Tweedie distribution, respectively.

10

Binary and count outcomes

The case of mixed binary and count responses is particularly relevant in clinical research, where the simultaneous prediction of health metrics helps evaluate the quality of care and performance indicators [Lingsma et al., 2018, Han et al., 2022]. Commonly used outcomes include in-hospital mortality, length of stay and readmission rates. These variables are inherently interrelated, which necessitates joint modeling.

This chapter illustrates the application of the copula regression approach to hospital data, focusing on modeling the relationship between length of stay and mortality risk. Joint regression allows for a deeper understanding of the variables driving these clinical metrics, enabling more comprehensive risk assessments and guiding patient management strategies.

10.1 Hospital length of stay and mortality

The framework is illustrated using data on in-hospital length of stay (`los`) and mortality (`died`), collected from patients admitted between January and September 2014 to Lewis Gale Medical Center, an over-500-bed facility in the state of Virginia [Azadeh-Fard et al., 2016]. The available regressors are `age`, `gender`, `bmi`, variables measuring vital signs, specifically temperature (`temp`), `pulse`, `respiratory` rate, `sbp` (systolic blood pressure) and `avpu` score (patient's level of consciousness), physiological measures, namely `dbp` (diastolic blood pressure) and `spO2` (oxygen saturation level), and subjective assessments on `severity` level and `risk` of dying. The dataset contains 978 observations.

In-hospital length of stay is generally linked to mortality, as patients with severe conditions or complications tend to remain hospitalized longer and face an increased risk of dying. However, prolonged hospitalization can also be associated with fewer deaths, as it allows for closer monitoring and comprehensive treatment, improving outcomes for some patients. Joint regression modeling provides a deeper understanding of the relationships between the aforementioned health outcomes and the impact of risk factors on them, enabling more effective assessments of health risks in patients with varying profiles.

10.2 Model

Let us consider a pair of random variables (Y_1, Y_2), where $Y_1 \sim \text{Ber}(\mu_1)$, $Y_2 \sim D_2(\mu_2, \sigma_2)$ is specified using any of the distributions reported in Table 1.2, $g_{\mu_1}(\mu_1) = \eta_{\mu_1}(\boldsymbol{x}_{\mu_1}; \boldsymbol{\beta}_{\mu_1})$, $\log(\mu_2) = \eta_{\mu_2}(\boldsymbol{x}_{\mu_2}; \boldsymbol{\beta}_{\mu_2})$ and $\log(\sigma_2) = \eta_{\sigma_2}(\boldsymbol{x}_{\sigma_2}; \boldsymbol{\beta}_{\sigma_2})$.

The joint CDF of Y_1 and Y_2 can be represented as

$$\mathbb{P}(Y_1 = 0, \ Y_2 \leq y_2) = C(F_1(0; \mu_1), \ F_2(y_2; \mu_2, \sigma_2); \theta),$$

where $F_1(0; \mu_1)$ and $F_2(y_2; \mu_2, \sigma_2)$ are the marginal CDFs of Y_1 evaluated at 0 and Y_2, respectively, and $C(\cdot, \cdot; \theta)$ is a copula function with dependence parameter that can be specified as $g_\theta(\theta) = \eta_\theta(\boldsymbol{x}_\theta; \boldsymbol{\beta}_\theta)$.

Using the fact that $f_2(y_2; \mu_2, \sigma_2) = F_2(y_2; \mu_2, \sigma_2) - F_2(y_2 - 1; \mu_2, \sigma_2)$, the joint PMF can be written as

$$\begin{aligned}
f_{12}(y_1, y_2; \mu_1, \mu_2, \sigma_2, \theta) = &\{C\left(F_1(0; \mu_1), F_2(y_2; \mu_2, \sigma_2); \theta\right) \\
&- C\left(F_1(0; \mu_1), F_2(y_2; \mu_2, \sigma_2) - f_2(y_2; \mu_2, \sigma_2); \theta\right)\}^{1-y_1} \\
&+ \{f_2(y_2; \mu_2, \sigma_2) - C\left(F_1(0; \mu_1), F_2(y_2; \mu_2, \sigma_2); \theta\right) \\
&+ C\left(F_1(0; \mu_1), F_2(y_2; \mu_2, \sigma_2) - f_2(y_2; \mu_2, \sigma_2); \theta\right)\}^{y_1}
\end{aligned}, \quad (10.1)$$

where $f_2(y_2; \mu_2, \sigma_2)$ is the marginal PMF of Y_2.

10.3 Log-likelihood

Using equation (10.1), for a random sample $(y_{i1}, y_{i2}, \boldsymbol{x}_i)_{i=1}^n$, where the covariate vector $\boldsymbol{x}_i$ is the union of $\boldsymbol{x}_{i\mu_1}$, $\boldsymbol{x}_{i\mu_2}$, $\boldsymbol{x}_{i\sigma_2}$ and $\boldsymbol{x}_{i\theta}$, the log-likelihood of the mixed binary and count outcomes copula regression model is

$$\begin{aligned}
\ell(\boldsymbol{\beta}) = \sum_{i=1}^n [&(1 - y_{i1}) \log \{C\left(F_1(0; \mu_{i1}), F_2(y_{i2}; \mu_{i2}, \sigma_{i2}); \theta_i\right) \\
&- C\left(F_1(0; \mu_{i1}), F_2(y_{i2}; \mu_{i2}, \sigma_{i2}) - f_2(y_{i2}; \mu_{i2}, \sigma_{i2}); \theta_i\right)\} \\
&+ y_{i1} \log \{f_2(y_{i2}; \mu_{i2}, \sigma_{i2}) - C\left(F_1(0; \mu_{i1}), F_2(y_{i2}; \mu_{i2}, \sigma_{i2}); \theta_i\right) \\
&+ C\left(F_1(0; \mu_{i1}), F_2(y_{i2}; \mu_{i2}, \sigma_{i2}) - f_2(y_{i2}; \mu_{i2}, \sigma_{i2}); \theta_i\right)\}]
\end{aligned},$$

where $\boldsymbol{\beta} = (\boldsymbol{\beta}_{\mu_1}^\top, \boldsymbol{\beta}_{\mu_2}^\top, \boldsymbol{\beta}_{\sigma_2}^\top, \boldsymbol{\beta}_\theta^\top)^\top$ is the overall regression coefficient vector.

10.4 Model fitting

Various models were evaluated, featuring a range of copulae, different link functions for the Bernoulli parameter and zero-truncated count distributions (since the length of stay only takes values greater than 0). Several specifications for the additive predictors of the distributional parameters were also considered. Based on convergence and residual checks, parsimony, information-based criteria and the *edf* values for the smooths of `age`, `bmi`, `sp02`, `sbp`, `dbp`, `pulse`, `respiratory` and `temp`, the preferred model is

```
library(GJRM); library(GJRM.data)
data(hospital)
```

```
eq1 <- died ~ age + gender + bmi + severity + risk + sp02 + sbp +
             dbp + pulse + respiratory + avpu + temp
eq2 <- los  ~ s(age) + gender + bmi + severity + risk + sp02 + sbp +
             dbp + pulse + respiratory + avpu + temp
eq3 <-      ~ age + gender + bmi + severity + risk + sp02 + sbp +
             dbp + pulse + respiratory + avpu + temp
eq4 <-      ~ 1
out <- gjrm(list(eq1, eq2, eq3, eq4), data = hospital,
            margin = c("logit", "tNBI"), copula = "T", model = "B")
```

where only one smooth term is kept in the model and θ is not influenced by covariate effects.

```
conv.check(out)
```

```
##
## Maximum absolute gradient value: 4.237606e-06
## Observed information matrix is positive definite
```

```
res.check(out, intervals = TRUE)
```

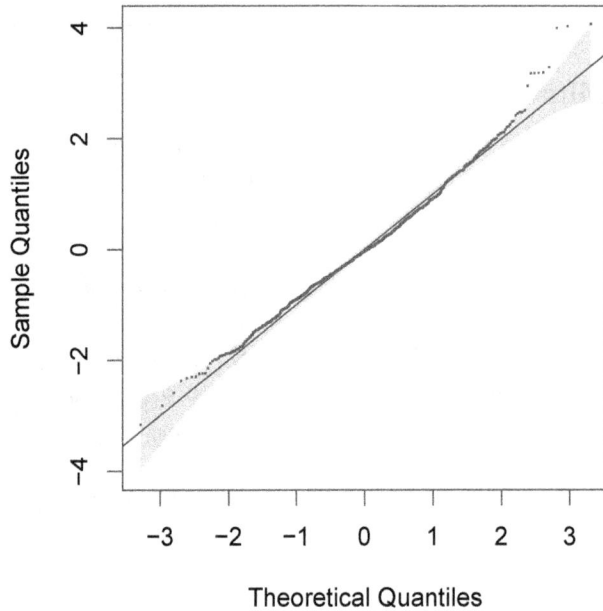

FIGURE 10.1 Normal Q–Q plot of randomized normalized quantile residuals for the count outcome, derived from a Student-t copula additive distributional regression model with `logit` and `tNBI` margins fitted to the `hospital` data.

Convergence checks are satisfactory, and the residual plot displayed in Figure 10.1 supports the choice of marginal count distribution.

The results are outlined in the outputs and comments that follow.

`summary(out)`

```
## 
## COPULA: Student-t
## MARGIN 1: Bernoulli
## MARGIN 2: Truncated Negative Binomial - Type I
## 
## EQUATION 1
## Link function for mu1: logit
## Formula: died ~ age + gender + bmi + severity + risk + sp02 + sbp + dbp
##     + pulse + respiratory + avpu + temp
## 
## Parametric coefficients:
##                       Estimate Std. Error z value Pr(>|z|)
## (Intercept)          13.113420  17.635763   0.744   0.4571
## age                   0.023483   0.015420   1.523   0.1278
## genderM               0.732617   0.414830   1.766   0.0774 .
## bmi                  -0.050473   0.034703  -1.454   0.1458
## severity2 - Moderate -0.116799   1.271182  -0.092   0.9268
## severity3 - Major     1.278882   1.328356   0.963   0.3357
## severity4 - Extreme   1.743321   1.419377   1.228   0.2194
## risk2 - Moderate     -0.245974   1.065383  -0.231   0.8174
## risk3 - Major         0.802365   1.090948   0.735   0.4621
## risk4 - Extreme       1.998690   1.180786   1.693   0.0905 .
## sp02                 -0.099347   0.049280  -2.016   0.0438 *
## sbp                  -0.005454   0.010260  -0.532   0.5950
## dbp                   0.011558   0.015234   0.759   0.4480
## pulse                 0.003824   0.010174   0.376   0.7070
## respiratory           0.058869   0.039521   1.490   0.1363
## avpuP                 0.885358   1.249522   0.709   0.4786
## avpuU                 1.974280   0.840269   2.350   0.0188 *
## avpuV                -0.776597   1.046821  -0.742   0.4582
## temp                 -0.109637   0.164572  -0.666   0.5053
## ---
## Signif. codes:  0 '***' 0.001 '**' 0.01 '*' 0.05 '.' 0.1 ' ' 1
## 
## 
## EQUATION 2
## Link function for mu2: log
## Formula: los ~ s(age) + gender + bmi + severity + risk + sp02 + sbp +
##     dbp + pulse + respiratory + avpu + temp
## 
## Parametric coefficients:
##                       Estimate Std. Error z value Pr(>|z|)
## (Intercept)          -1.720568   2.954199  -0.582 0.560287
## genderM              -0.192465   0.054275  -3.546 0.000391 ***
## bmi                   0.001824   0.004345   0.420 0.674691
## severity2 - Moderate  0.372561   0.098216   3.793 0.000149 ***
## severity3 - Major     0.693571   0.118094   5.873 4.28e-09 ***
## severity4 - Extreme   1.258014   0.173944   7.232 4.75e-13 ***
```

```
## risk2 - Moderate      0.177076   0.081373   2.176 0.029548 *
## risk3 - Major         0.245065   0.103718   2.363 0.018137 *
## risk4 - Extreme       0.246318   0.183074   1.345 0.178478
## sp02                  0.010183   0.007986   1.275 0.202283
## sbp                  -0.000479   0.001363  -0.352 0.725209
## dbp                  -0.003510   0.002244  -1.564 0.117786
## pulse                 0.002570   0.001524   1.686 0.091793 .
## respiratory          -0.003652   0.010213  -0.358 0.720638
## avpuP                -0.020031   0.493273  -0.041 0.967608
## avpuU                -0.391983   0.364142  -1.076 0.281722
## avpuV                -0.102432   0.167315  -0.612 0.540396
## temp                  0.017443   0.028294   0.617 0.537562
## ---
## Signif. codes:  0 '***' 0.001 '**' 0.01 '*' 0.05 '.' 0.1 ' ' 1
##
## Approximate significance of smooth terms:
##           edf Ref.df Chi.sq p-value
## s(age) 3.014  3.791  13.62 0.00825 **
## ---
## Signif. codes:  0 '***' 0.001 '**' 0.01 '*' 0.05 '.' 0.1 ' ' 1
##
##
## sigma2 = 0.422(0.169,1.21)
## theta = -0.574(-0.711,-0.379)
## n = 978   total edf = 60
```

The estimated correlation is negative and significant, suggesting an inverse dependence between the probability of dying and the length of hospital stay. This indicates that patients who stay in the hospital longer tend to have a lower likelihood of dying, possibly because of the need for extended recovery or ongoing treatment. In contrast, patients with shorter hospital stays may face a higher risk of dying, potentially due to rapid health deterioration or premature death.

Variables gender, sp02 and avpu have a significant impact on the propensity of dying. In particular, male patients have twice the odds of dying compared to female patients, while higher oxygen saturation levels are associated with a lower probability of dying. Regarding avpu, the odds of death for unresponsive patients are approximately seven times higher than those who are fully alert. This dramatic difference highlights the crucial role of consciousness level in influencing mortality.

Regarding the count outcome, gender, severity, risk and age emerge as strong predictors. Broadly speaking, male patients tend to have shorter hospital stays than females, while more severe and risky cases require significantly longer hospital stays, highlighting how critical conditions drive resource utilization due to intensive care needs. As shown in Figure 10.2, the length of stay increases as patients age, peaking around 70, before gradually declining in older age groups. This pattern may indicate that middle-aged and young elderly patients require extended care due to age-related issues, while very elderly patients may experience shorter stays, possibly due to higher mortality rates leading to early discharge. Alternatively, the shorter stays in older age groups could be related to different healthcare strategies, such as a focus on palliative care. The results for σ_2 (not shown here) indicate that risk and age are the primary regressors influencing this parameter.

```
plot(out, eq = 2, rug = TRUE, jit = TRUE)
```

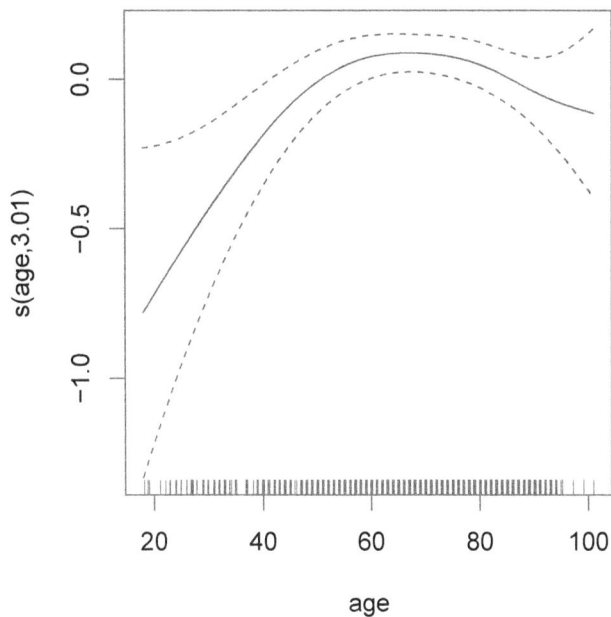

FIGURE 10.2 Estimated smooth effect (with associated 95% intervals) of `age` on the scale of the additive predictor of μ_2, derived from a Student-t copula additive distributional regression model with `logit` and `tNBI` margins fitted to the `hospital` data.

The effects that the covariates have on the length of stay can be quantified by predicting the average in-hospital duration for given patient characteristics.

```
nd <- nd1 <- data.frame(age = 68, gender = "F", bmi = 28,
                        risk = "1 - Minor", sp02 = 97, sbp = 135, dbp = 73,
                        pulse = 81,  respiratory = 18, avpu = "A", temp = 98,
                        severity = "1 - Minor")
nd1$severity <- "4 - Extreme"

marg.mv(out, eq = 2, newdata = nd)

##
## Marginal mean with 95% interval:
##
## 3.14 (2.83,3.54)

marg.mv(out, eq = 2, newdata = nd1)

##
## Marginal mean with 95% interval:
##
## 10.40 (7.98,16.60)
```

When severity is minor, the marginal mean of `los` is predicted to be approximately three days, with a relatively narrow interval. For an extreme severity level, the predicted mean increases sharply to around 10 and a half days. However, this is accompanied by a wide interval, likely due to greater variability in hospitalization durations at this severity level.

Joint and conditional probabilities are given by (10.1), and the ratio of (10.1) to the marginal PMF on which the probability is conditioned. Some examples are presented in the following outputs.

```
nd <- data.frame(age = 68, gender = "F", bmi = 28,
                 severity = "2 - Moderate",  risk = "1 - Minor",
                 sp02 = 97, sbp = 135, dbp = 73, pulse = 81,
                 respiratory = 18, avpu = "A", temp = 98)

copula.prob(out, y1 = 0, y2 = 1, newdata = nd, intervals = TRUE)

##          p12       2.5%       97.5%
##   0.1655609 0.1173798 0.2005316

copula.prob(out, y1 = 1, y2 = 1, newdata = nd, cond = 2, intervals = TRUE)

##          p12        2.5%       97.5%
##   0.01603149 0.003499718 0.1170329

copula.prob(out, y1 = 1, y2 = 3, newdata = nd, cond = 2, intervals = TRUE)

##          p12         2.5%        97.5%
##   0.0003664819 3.984292e-05 0.003121857
```

The model predicts a joint probability of 16.6% that this patient will both survive and have a hospital stay of one day. The probability of dying decreases from 1.6% after one day in the hospital to 0.04% after three days, suggesting that longer hospitalizations are linked to a significantly lower mortality risk.

Conditional expectations offer additional insights and are defined as

$$\mathbb{E}(Y_2|Y_1 = 0) = \frac{1}{F_1(0;\mu_1)} \sum_{y_2=1}^{\infty} y_2 f_{12}(0, y_2; \mu_1, \mu_2, \sigma_1, \sigma_2, \theta),$$

and similarly for $\mathbb{E}(Y_2|Y_1 = 1)$. The upper bound of the summation is set to a specified value, ensuring that terms beyond this point contribute negligibly to the overall sum. Intervals are conveniently obtained through posterior simulation.

```
cond.mv(out, eq = 2, y1 = 0, newdata = nd)

##
## Conditional mean with 95% interval:
##
## 4.11 (3.71,4.60)

cond.mv(out, eq = 2, y1 = 1, newdata = nd)

##
## Conditional mean with 95% interval:
##
## 2.20 (1.61,3.99)
```

Patients who survive have an expected hospital stay of approximately four days, while those who do not survive have shorter stays, averaging about two days. These findings provide helpful insights for guiding resource allocation within the hospital.

Future research will focus on developing a trivariate regression model to jointly examine in-hospital length of stay, mortality and readmission rates.

11

Count and continuous outcomes

Jointly modeling of mixed count and continuous outcomes is essential in various fields of study. In non-life insurance, for example, simultaneously analyzing the number and size of claims provides valuable insights for risk assessment and premium setting [Lu, 2019]. In medicine, examining the frequency and duration of physical activity offers a more comprehensive understanding of health behaviors and their effects on well-being [Siddique et al., 2023]. In toxicity research, modeling both malformations and fetal weight helps identify the underlying variables contributing to developmental abnormalities [Catalano and Ryan, 1992].

Copula regression models for count and continuous outcomes, as developed by Marra and Radice [2025b], are explored here with an emphasis on jointly analyzing the number and cost of physician visits. The approach provides a more comprehensive view of how these outcomes interact and how covariates impact them, offering meaningful insights into patient behavior patterns.

11.1 Number and cost of visits to physicians

The modeling technique is illustrated using the MEPS data introduced in Chapter 3. The aim is to jointly model the number and cost of visits to physicians conditional on covariate information. The outcomes are `dvisit` (number of consultations with a doctor) and `dvexpend` (expenditure on doctor visits). When no visits occur, both responses are equal to zero, resulting in a lack of variability that hinders the study of the underlying mechanisms driving them. Therefore, zeros are excluded from the analysis. The available covariates are `bmi`, `income`, `age`, `gender`, `ethnicity`, `education`, `region`, `hypertension` and `hyperlipidemia`.

The relationship between visit frequency and costs is complex and often nonlinear. For instance, chronic conditions may require frequent, low-cost visits, while surgeries or specialized care involve fewer but higher-cost treatments. Jointly modeling captures this complexity, providing a clearer understanding of how visit frequency influences costs and vice versa, which is essential for effective healthcare planning. Moreover, the approach can shed light on the variables influencing healthcare utilization and expenses simultaneously, revealing nuanced patient behaviors and assisting in the development of cost-effective strategies while maintaining quality of care.

DOI: 10.1201/9781003593195-11

11.2   Model

Let us define Y_1 and Y_2 as the random variables representing count and continuous responses which can follow any of the distributions listed in Tables 1.2 and 1.3, respectively. The joint CDF of Y_1 and Y_2 can be represented as

$$\mathbb{P}(Y_1 \leq y_1,\ Y_2 \leq y_2) = C(F_1(y_1; \mu_1, \sigma_1),\ F_2(y_2; \mu_2, \sigma_2, \nu_2); \theta),$$

where $F_1(y_1; \mu_1, \sigma_1)$ and $F_2(y_2; \mu_2, \sigma_2, \nu_2)$ are the marginal CDFs of Y_1 and Y_2, $g_{\mu_j}(\mu_j) = \eta_{\mu_j}(\boldsymbol{x}_{\mu_j}; \boldsymbol{\beta}_{\mu_j})$ and $g_{\sigma_j}(\sigma_j) = \eta_{\sigma_j}(\boldsymbol{x}_{\sigma_j}; \boldsymbol{\beta}_{\sigma_j})$, for $j = 1, 2$, $g_{\nu_2}(\nu_2) = \eta_{\nu_2}(\boldsymbol{x}_{\nu_2}; \boldsymbol{\beta}_{\mu_2})$ and $C(\cdot, \cdot; \theta)$ is a copula function with dependence parameter specified as $g_\theta(\theta) = \eta_\theta(\boldsymbol{x}_\theta; \boldsymbol{\beta}_\theta)$.

Using the fact that $f_1(y_1; \mu_1, \sigma_1) = F_1(y_1; \mu_1, \sigma_1) - F_1(y_1 - 1; \mu_1, \sigma_1)$, the joint PDF is formulated as

$$
\begin{aligned}
f_{12}(y_1, y_2; \mu_1, \mu_2, \sigma_1, \sigma_2, \nu_2, \theta) =\, & f_2(y_2; \mu_2, \sigma_2, \nu_2) \left[\frac{\partial C\left(F_1(y_1; \mu_1, \sigma_1), F_2(y_2; \mu_2, \sigma_2, \nu_2); \theta\right)}{\partial \partial F_2(y_2; \mu_2, \sigma_2, \nu_2)} \right. \\
& \left. - \frac{\partial C\left(F_1(y_1; \mu_1, \sigma_1) - f_1(y_1; \mu_1, \sigma_1), F_2(y_2; \mu_2, \sigma_2, \nu_2); \theta\right)}{\partial \partial F_2(y_2; \mu_2, \sigma_2, \nu_2)} \right],
\end{aligned}
$$

(11.1)

where $f_1(y_1; \mu_1, \sigma_1)$ and $f_2(y_2; \mu_2, \sigma_2, \nu_2)$ are the marginals PMF and PDF of Y_1 and Y_2.

The joint probability $\mathbb{P}(Y_1 = y_1, Y_2 \leq y_2)$ is defined as

$$
\begin{aligned}
\mathbb{P}(Y_1 = y_1, Y_2 \leq y_2) =\, & C\left(F_1(y_1; \mu_1, \sigma_1), F_2(y_2; \mu_2, \sigma_2, \nu_2); \theta\right) \\
& - C\left(F_1(y_1; \mu_1, \sigma_1) - f_1(y_1; \mu_1, \sigma_1), F_2(y_2; \mu_2, \sigma_2, \nu_2); \theta\right),
\end{aligned}
$$

(11.2)

whereas the conditional probabilities $\mathbb{P}(Y_1 = y_1 | Y_2 = y_2)$ and $\mathbb{P}(Y_2 \leq y_2 | Y_1 = y_1)$ are given by the ratio of (11.1) and $f_2(y_2; \mu_2, \sigma_2, \nu_2)$, and the ratio of (11.2) and $f_1(y_1; \mu_1, \sigma_1)$, respectively.

11.3   Log-likelihood

Using equation (11.1), for a random sample $(y_{i1}, y_{i2}, \boldsymbol{x}_i)_{i=1}^{n}$, where the covariate vector $\boldsymbol{x}_i$ is the union of $\boldsymbol{x}_{i\mu_1}$, $\boldsymbol{x}_{i\mu_2}$, $\boldsymbol{x}_{i\sigma_1}$, $\boldsymbol{x}_{i\sigma_2}$, $\boldsymbol{x}_{i\nu_2}$ and $\boldsymbol{x}_{i\theta}$, the log-likelihood of the mixed count and continuous outcomes copula regression model is

$$\ell(\boldsymbol{\beta}) = \sum_{i=1}^{n} \log \left\{ f_{12}(y_{i1}, y_{i2}; \mu_{i1}, \mu_{i2}, \sigma_{i1}, \sigma_{i2}, \nu_{i2}, \theta_i) \right\},$$

where $\boldsymbol{\beta} = (\boldsymbol{\beta}_{\mu_1}^\top, \boldsymbol{\beta}_{\mu_2}^\top, \boldsymbol{\beta}_{\sigma_1}^\top, \boldsymbol{\beta}_{\sigma_2}^\top, \boldsymbol{\beta}_{\nu_2}^\top, \boldsymbol{\beta}_\theta^\top)^\top$ is the overall regression coefficient vector.

11.4   Model fitting

Various combinations of copulae, marginal distributions (specifically, zero-truncated count and continuous distributions with positive support) and additive predictors for all the distributional parameters were considered. Based on convergence diagnostics, residual checks, parsimony and information-based criteria, as well as the estimated shapes for the smooth terms of `bmi`, `income`, `age` and `education`, the preferred model is

```
library(GJRM); library(GJRM.data)
data(meps); meps1 <- meps[meps$dvisit > 0,]

eq1 <- dvisit   ~ bmi + income + age + education + ethnicity + region +
                  gender + hypertension + hyperlipidemia
eq2 <- dvexpend ~ bmi + income + s(age) + education + ethnicity + region +
                  gender + hypertension + hyperlipidemia

out <- gjrm(list(eq1, eq2), margins = c("tNBII", "DAGUM"), copula = "G180",
            model = "B", data = meps1, uni.fit = TRUE)
conv.check(out)
```

```
##
## Maximum absolute gradient value: 0.001345943
## Observed information matrix is positive definite
```

Convergence checks are adequate, and the residual plots reported in Figure 11.1 generally support the choice of marginal distributions, despite some lack of fit with the `DAGUM`.

```
res.check(out, intervals = TRUE)
```

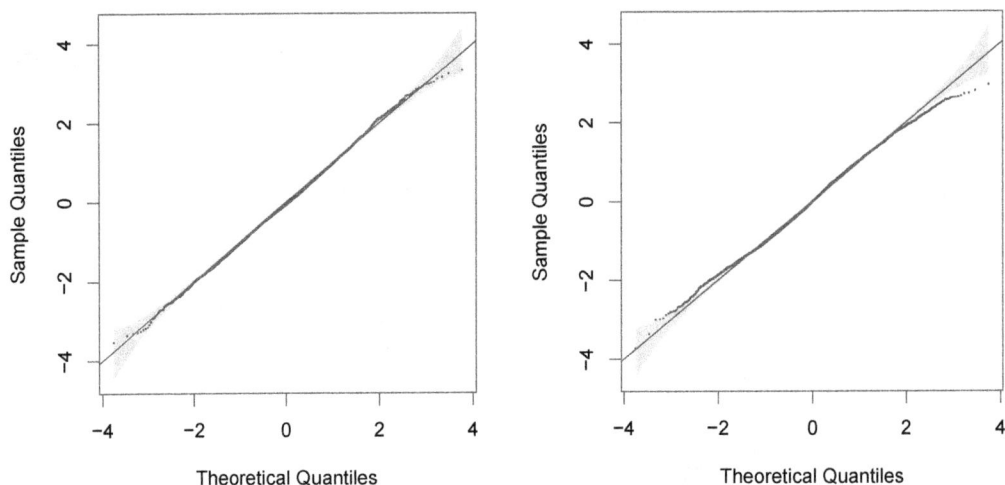

FIGURE 11.1 Normal Q–Q plot of normalized quantile residuals, derived from a 180° rotated Gumbel copula additive distributional regression model with `tNBII` and `DAGUM` margins fitted to the `meps1` data.

A detailed examination of the results follows.

summary(out)

```
##
## COPULA: 180° Gumbel
## MARGIN 1: Truncated Negative Binomial - Type II
## MARGIN 2: Dagum
##
## EQUATION 1
## Link function for mu1: log
## Formula: dvisit ~ bmi + income + age + education + ethnicity + region +
##     gender + hypertension + hyperlipidemia
##
## Parametric coefficients:
##                Estimate Std. Error z value Pr(>|z|)
## (Intercept)   -1.093e+00  2.288e-01  -4.777 1.78e-06 ***
## bmi            1.684e-02  3.459e-03   4.869 1.12e-06 ***
## income        -2.499e-06  7.125e-07  -3.507 0.000453 ***
## age            2.223e-02  2.879e-03   7.722 1.14e-14 ***
## education      4.335e-02  9.748e-03   4.448 8.68e-06 ***
## ethnicity2    -1.556e-01  6.277e-02  -2.478 0.013203 *
## ethnicity3    -1.336e-01  2.628e-01  -0.508 0.611295
## ethnicity4    -2.766e-01  1.246e-01  -2.219 0.026461 *
## region2       -8.331e-03  7.496e-02  -0.111 0.911508
## region3       -7.080e-02  6.912e-02  -1.024 0.305666
## region4       -1.439e-01  8.116e-02  -1.773 0.076261 .
## gender        -3.319e-01  5.662e-02  -5.863 4.55e-09 ***
## hypertension   2.355e-01  6.443e-02   3.655 0.000257 ***
## hyperlipidemia 3.201e-01  6.121e-02   5.229 1.71e-07 ***
## ---
## Signif. codes:  0 '***' 0.001 '**' 0.01 '*' 0.05 '.' 0.1 ' ' 1
##
##
## EQUATION 2
## Link function for mu2: log
## Formula: dvexpend ~ bmi + income + s(age) + education + ethnicity + region
##     + gender + hypertension + hyperlipidemia
##
## Parametric coefficients:
##                Estimate Std. Error z value Pr(>|z|)
## (Intercept)    4.831e+00  1.231e-01  39.263  < 2e-16 ***
## bmi            3.215e-03  2.254e-03   1.427  0.15369
## income        -3.057e-09  3.108e-07  -0.010  0.99215
## education      3.779e-02  5.393e-03   7.008 2.42e-12 ***
## ethnicity2    -6.594e-02  3.646e-02  -1.809  0.07053 .
## ethnicity3    -1.996e-02  1.451e-01  -0.138  0.89059
## ethnicity4    -1.593e-01  5.241e-02  -3.040  0.00237 **
## region2        2.000e-02  4.518e-02   0.443  0.65790
## region3       -1.126e-01  4.098e-02  -2.747  0.00602 **
## region4       -3.007e-02  4.463e-02  -0.674  0.50051
```

```
## gender          -1.532e-01  2.989e-02  -5.126 2.96e-07 ***
## hypertension      9.753e-02  3.726e-02   2.618  0.00885 **
## hyperlipidemia    1.836e-01  3.641e-02   5.042 4.60e-07 ***
## ---
## Signif. codes:  0 '***' 0.001 '**' 0.01 '*' 0.05 '.' 0.1 ' ' 1
##
## Approximate significance of smooth terms:
##          edf Ref.df Chi.sq p-value
## s(age) 2.464  3.099  80.31  <2e-16 ***
## ---
## Signif. codes:  0 '***' 0.001 '**' 0.01 '*' 0.05 '.' 0.1 ' ' 1
##
## sigma1 = 4.43(4.14,4.73)  sigma2 = 1.25(1.21,1.3)
## nu2 = 1.49(1.33,1.63)
## theta = 2.64(2.56,2.71)
## n = 5752  total edf = 33.5

plot(out, eq = 2, rug = TRUE, jit = TRUE)
```

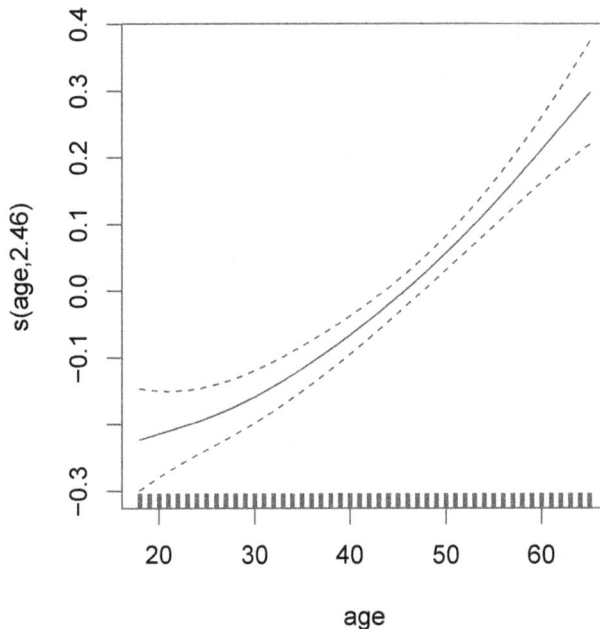

FIGURE 11.2 Estimated smooth effect (with associated 95% intervals) of age on the scale of the additive predictor of μ_2, derived from a 180° rotated Gumbel copula additive distributional regression model with tNBII and DAGUM margins fitted to the meps1 data.

Higher values of bmi lead to more frequent visits, likely due to the increased risk of health issues, such as diabetes and cardiovascular diseases, associated with elevated bmi. Higher income is associated with fewer doctor visits, yet income does not seem to influence the expenditure on those visits. This indicates that while wealthier individuals may access healthcare less frequently, possibly due to better overall health or preventive care, the cost per visit remains relatively constant regardless of income. Older individuals tend to visit doctors more frequently, probably because of the increased prevalence of medical conditions associated with aging that require regular monitoring. As shown in Figure 11.2, costs generally increase with `age` but at varying rates, thus reflecting the different levels of medical care required at different life stages. Higher `education` levels are associated with more frequent doctor visits and potentially higher healthcare costs. This could be attributed to better health literacy and a stronger focus on preventive healthcare among more educated individuals, as well as greater access to health insurance. The variable `ethnicity` affects healthcare usage and costs, with different patterns emerging across ethnic groups, potentially due to variations in healthcare access and cultural attitudes. The `region` in which an individual resides influences healthcare costs, though not necessarily the frequency of visits. For example, living in the South is associated with lower expenditures compared to living in the Northeast, potentially due to regional pricing differences, availability of services or local policies. Females tend to visit doctors more frequently and incur higher associated costs than males, reflecting gender-specific needs and behaviors. The presence of chronic conditions such as `hypertension` and `hyperlipidemia` leads to more frequent doctor visits and higher costs due to the ongoing need for monitoring, treatment and management.

The copula parameter captures a positive dependence between `dvisit` and `dvexpend`, suggesting the presence of underlying variables, such as individual health behaviors, psychological factors and healthcare literacy, that may influence the outcomes.

Covariate effects can be quantified through prediction.

```
nd <- nd1 <- data.frame(bmi = 27, income = 52000, age = 44, education = 13,
                        gender = 0, ethnicity = 1, region = 3,
                        hypertension = 0, hyperlipidemia = 0)
nd1$hyperlipidemia <- 1

marg.mv(out, eq = 1, newdata = nd)

##
## Marginal mean with 95% interval:
##
## 3.76 (3.61,3.92)

marg.mv(out, eq = 1, newdata = nd1)

##
## Marginal mean with 95% interval:
##
## 4.25 (4.05,4.55)
```

The example above shows the impact of `hyperlipidemia` on the expected number of doctor visits for a typical subject. As expected, an individual with hyperlipidemia has a higher number of doctor visits compared to the same individual without the condition.

Other measures of interest are conditional expectations. For the continuous outcome, this is defined as

$$\mathbb{E}(Y_2|Y_1 = y_1) = \frac{1}{f_1(y_1; \mu_1, \sigma_1)} \int y_2 f_{12}(y_1, y_2; \mu_1, \mu_2, \sigma_1, \sigma_2, \nu_2, \theta) dy_2,$$

where the integration is over the support of y_2 and intervals are conveniently obtained through posterior simulation. For a typical patient, the average expenditures given one and four doctor visits are displayed below.

```
cond.mv(out, eq = 2, y1 = 1, newdata = nd)
```

```
##
## Conditional mean with 95% interval:
##
## 146 (137,154)
```

```
cond.mv(out, eq = 2, y1 = 4, newdata = nd)
```

```
##
## Conditional mean with 95% interval:
##
## 815 (764,870)
```

The estimates reveal a significant increase in healthcare expenditure as the number of doctor visits rises, with the cost disparity between one and four visits highlighting the impact of visit frequency.

For the count outcome, the conditional expectation is

$$\mathbb{E}(Y_1|Y_2 = y_2) = \frac{1}{f_2(y_2; \mu_2, \sigma_2, \nu_2)} \sum_{y_1=1}^{\infty} y_1 f_{12}(y_1, y_2; \mu_1, \mu_2, \sigma_1, \sigma_2, \nu_2, \theta),$$

where the summation is approximated using an upper bound selected to ensure that terms beyond this value contribute negligibly to the overall sum.

```
cond.mv(out, eq = 1, y2 = 100, newdata = nd)
```

```
##
## Conditional mean with 95% interval:
##
## 1.34 (1.30,1.39)
```

```
cond.mv(out, eq = 1, y2 = 800, newdata = nd)
```

```
##
## Conditional mean with 95% interval:
##
## 5.52 (5.37,5.70)
```

More frequent doctor visits are associated with higher spending, although the relationship is nonlinear. For a cost of \$100, the expected number of visits is approximately one day, increasing to about six days for \$800. This suggests that as costs rise, the frequency of visits increases at a diminishing rate, indicating a shift toward more expensive, intensive or specialized care.

Part IV

Copula Regression for Unobserved Confounding

12

Binary outcome with binary treatment effect

Assessing the causal effect of a treatment on an outcome can be challenging in observational studies due to nonrandom treatment allocation. This lack of randomization necessitates controlling for observed and unobserved confounders that may influence both the treatment and outcome. Similarly, in randomized controlled trials, nonadherence can undermine the validity of randomization by creating differences between groups that are influenced by confounders. If these are not accounted for, inconsistent estimates of the average treatment effect (ATE) are to be expected. This problem, commonly referred to as endogeneity of the treatment variable, is addressed here using the structural equation approach by Marra and Radice [2011]. For an overview of standard and more specialized causal frameworks, see Freedman [2009] and Clarke and Windmeijer [2012].

The approach is employed to analyze a dataset from a reemployment experiment, aiming to isolate the causal effect of a cash bonus on the probability of finding a job.

12.1   Illinois reemployment experiment

The case study revisits the Illinois Reemployment Bonus Experiment, conducted by the Illinois Department of Employment Security between mid-1984 and mid-1985, which aimed to examine the effect of a cash bonus on the duration of insured unemployment [Woodbury and Spiegelman, 1987]. In this experiment, eligible beneficiaries of unemployment insurance were randomly allocated to one of three groups: the Job Search Incentive Experiment group, the Hiring Incentive Experiment group (HIE) or the control group. This analysis focuses on the HIE group, where companies could claim the bonus by hiring job seekers within 11 weeks of the start of their unemployment spells, provided the jobs lasted over 30 hours per week for at least four months. The dataset includes a total of 7,734 observations.

While group allocation was randomized, the decision to participate in the experiment was not. Specifically, the treatment variable `agree` is equal to 1 if an individual was assigned to the HIE group and agreed to participate, or 0 if they were assigned to the control group or chose not to participate. The binary indicator for group or bonus assignment, `bonus`, is used as an instrument. This type of participation suggests that individual choices, most likely influenced by unobserved variables such as motivation, financial need and job prospects, may affect both the decision to participate and the probability of reemployment (or the duration of unemployment). For instance, individuals experiencing financial hardship might be more inclined to agree to participate in the experiment, yet their financial struggles could hinder their job-seeking efforts, prolonging unemployment or reducing their chances of reemployment. Similarly, those with low motivation may enroll in the experiment but fail to actively seek employment opportunities. Conversely, those opting out of the program may have better job prospects or higher motivation levels, which may shorten unemployment duration (or increase the probability of reemployment). The model discussed in this chapter addresses the issue of endogenous participation, thus helping isolate the causal effect of the bonus from both observed and unobserved confounding.

Following Bijwaard and Ridder [2005], the observed confounders include `age`, pre-unemployment earnings (`prearn`), `gender`, `ethnicity` and the weekly amount of unemployment insurance benefits plus dependence allowance (`benefit`). The follow-up time `unemp.dur` represents the duration of unemployment in weeks and is used as the outcome in the causal survival model discussed in Section 13.4. The `status` variable indicates whether an individual was reemployed within 26 weeks and serves as both the primary outcome variable for this study and the censoring indicator in the causal survival analysis in Section 13.4. Since unemployment insurance was provided for a maximum of 26 weeks, participants were observed only until the end of their claim period, leading to right-censoring at 26 weeks.

12.2   Model

Consider a pair of binary random variables (Y_1, Y_2), both following Bernoulli distributions. Specifically, $Y_1 \sim \mathrm{Ber}(\mu_1)$ with $g_{\mu_1}(\mu_1) = \eta_{\mu_1}(\boldsymbol{x}_{\mu_1}; \boldsymbol{\beta}_{\mu_1})$, where $\boldsymbol{x}_{\mu_1} = (\boldsymbol{x}_o^\top, \boldsymbol{x}_{iv}^\top)^\top$ contains observed confounders and at least an instrumental variable, and $\boldsymbol{\beta}_{\mu_1} = (\boldsymbol{\beta}_{o\mu_1}^\top, \boldsymbol{\beta}_{iv}^\top)^\top$. Similarly, $Y_2 \sim \mathrm{Ber}(\mu_2)$ with $g_{\mu_2}(\mu_2) = \eta_{\mu_2}(\boldsymbol{x}_{\mu_2}; \boldsymbol{\beta}_{\mu_2})$, where $\boldsymbol{x}_{\mu_2} = (\boldsymbol{x}_o^\top, y_1)^\top$ includes observed counfounders and the treatment, and $\boldsymbol{\beta}_{\mu_2} = (\boldsymbol{\beta}_{o\mu_2}^\top, \beta_{tr})^\top$. The model specification is completed by joining the CDFs of Y_1 and Y_2 via a copula function, as shown in equation (5.1). To achieve empirical identification, the instrumental variable(s) must be predictive of Y_1, not have a direct effect on Y_2 (exclusion restriction) and be independent of unobserved confounders (after accounting for observed confounders). This bivariate model is recursive, positing a direct effect of Y_1 on Y_2 but not vice versa. For treatment effect identification, the copula and marginal link functions are usually specified as Gaussian and probit, the assumptions adopted here. However, Han and Vytlacil [2017] proved identification under the general setting where the marginal distributions are arbitrary but known and C belongs to a broad class of parametric copulae, including those listed in Table 1.1.

The equations for Y_1 and Y_2 can be written as $Y_1^* = \eta_{\mu_1}(\boldsymbol{x}_{\mu_1}; \boldsymbol{\beta}_{\mu_1}) + \epsilon_1$ and $Y_2^* = \eta_{\mu_2}(\boldsymbol{x}_{\mu_2}; \boldsymbol{\beta}_{\mu_2}) + \epsilon_2$, where the error terms follow a standard bivariate Gaussian distribution with correlation ρ and $Y_j = \mathbf{1}\{Y_j^* > 0\}$, for $j = 1, 2$. This is helpful in illustrating the role of unobserved confounding from an omitted variable perspective. For example, the distribution of Y_2^* given $Y_1 = 1$ is Gaussian with mean

$$\eta_{\mu_2}\{(\boldsymbol{x}_{io}^\top, 1)^\top; \boldsymbol{\beta}_{\mu_2}\} + \rho \frac{\phi\left[\eta_{\mu_1}(\boldsymbol{x}_{\mu_1}; \boldsymbol{\beta}_{\mu_1})\right]}{\Phi\left[\eta_{\mu_1}(\boldsymbol{x}_{\mu_1}; \boldsymbol{\beta}_{\mu_1})\right]}$$

and variance

$$\rho^2 \left[-\eta_{\mu_1}(\boldsymbol{x}_{\mu_1}; \boldsymbol{\beta}_{\mu_1}) \frac{\phi\left[\eta_{\mu_1}(\boldsymbol{x}_{\mu_1}; \boldsymbol{\beta}_{\mu_1})\right]}{\Phi\left[\eta_{\mu_1}(\boldsymbol{x}_{\mu_1}; \boldsymbol{\beta}_{\mu_1})\right]} - \left(\frac{\phi\left[\eta_{\mu_1}(\boldsymbol{x}_{\mu_1}; \boldsymbol{\beta}_{\mu_1})\right]}{\Phi\left[\eta_{\mu_1}(\boldsymbol{x}_{\mu_1}; \boldsymbol{\beta}_{\mu_1})\right]} \right)^2 \right] + 1.$$

Similar expressions for the mean and variance are obtained for the distribution of Y_2^* given $Y_1 = 0$. These derivations indicate that fitting the outcome equation alone will result in inconsistent estimates when $\rho \neq 0$.

For an observed sample $(y_{i2}, \boldsymbol{x}_i)_{i=1}^n$, where $\boldsymbol{x}_i$ is the union of $\boldsymbol{x}_{i\mu_1}$ and $\boldsymbol{x}_{i\mu_2}$, the log-likelihood of the recursive bivariate binary model is given by (5.2).

12.3   Average treatment effect

The estimator of the ATE is

$$\mathrm{ATE}(\hat{\boldsymbol{\beta}}_{\mu_2}) = \frac{1}{n} \sum_{i=1}^n \left(\Phi\left[\eta_{\mu_2} \left\{ (\boldsymbol{x}_{io}^\top, 1)^\top ; \hat{\boldsymbol{\beta}}_{\mu_2} \right\} \right] - \Phi\left[\eta_{\mu_2} \left\{ (\boldsymbol{x}_{io}^\top, 0)^\top ; \hat{\boldsymbol{\beta}}_{\mu_2} \right\} \right] \right), \qquad (12.1)$$

with intervals conveniently obtained through posterior simulation.

12.4   Model fitting

The equations for μ_1 and μ_2, pertaining to the treatment and outcome agree and status, are specified as

```
library(GJRM); library(GJRM.data)
data(hie)

eq1 <- agree   ~ s(bonus, bs = "re") + age + prearn + benefit + gender +
                 ethnicity
eq2 <- status ~ agree*gender + s(age) + s(prearn) + benefit + ethnicity
fl  <- list(eq1, eq2)
```

Only the effects of age and prearn are estimated flexibly in the second equation. This choice was made because the additional smooth functions exhibited *edf* values close or equal to 1. The equation of interest includes an interaction term between agree and gender, with the latter considered an effect modifier. This allows for the examination of potential differences in job-seeking behavior between males and females.

```
table(hie$bonus, hie$agree)

##
##        0    1
##   0 3863    0
##   1 1340 2531
```

As shown in the table above, due to nonadherence, the values of bonus and agree may differ for the treated group, while for the control group, the two variables are identical since individuals cannot switch to the treatment. This may result in computational instability and a substantial increase in the variance of the estimator. To mitigate this issue, the approach discussed in Section 1.2.1 is employed, as reflected in the specification of eq1.

```
out <- gjrm(fl, data = hie, margins = c("probit", "probit"), model = "B")
conv.check(out)
```

```
##
## Maximum absolute gradient value: 3.819609e-07
## Observed information matrix is positive definite
```

```
summary(out, n.sim = 1000)
```

```
...
##
## theta = -0.0756(-0.157,0.00703)
## n = 7734   total edf = 17.8
```

Convergence checks are satisfactory, and the estimated correlation parameter is negative and only marginally not significant. This result supports the earlier explanation that unobserved confounders that increase the likelihood of individuals agreeing to participate in the experiment, also decrease their probability of reemployment. Failing to account for them will bias the treatment effect.

Below are the ATEs by gender using both the joint and univariate approaches, with the latter ignoring the issue of endogeneity.

```
ATE(out, trt = "agree", int.var = c("agree:gender", 0))
```

```
##
## Average treatment effect with 95% interval:
##
## 0.0285 (-0.0148,0.0737)
```

```
ATE(out, trt = "agree", int.var = c("agree:gender", 1))
```

```
##
## Average treatment effect with 95% interval:
##
## 0.0124 (-0.0226,0.0442)
```

```
ATE(out, trt = "agree", int.var = c("agree:gender", 0), joint = FALSE)
```

```
##
## Average treatment effect with 95% interval:
##
## 0.00734 (-0.01711,0.03310)
```

```
ATE(out, trt = "agree", int.var = c("agree:gender", 1), joint = FALSE)
```

```
##
## Average treatment effect with 95% interval:
##
## -0.0069 (-0.0325,0.0206)
```

None of the estimates are significantly different from zero, with those from the univariate approach being rather small. Despite the nonsignificance, looking at the results from the bivariate approach, a trend emerges: the cash bonus appears to be more important for females than for males. This could be attributed to gender-specific differences in job-seeking behavior, such as varying levels of urgency or motivation to secure employment. Moreover, women may face distinct barriers or incentives in the job market, making the bonus more impactful for them. Interpreting some of the effects, the probability of reemployment for females is 2.9 percentage points higher for individuals in the HIE group compared to the control group when accounting for unobserved confounders, whereas the probability increases by only 0.7 percentage points when neglecting them.

Additional results are discussed hereafter.

```
summary(out, n.sim = 1000)


##
## COPULA: Gaussian
## MARGIN 1: Bernoulli
## MARGIN 2: Bernoulli
##
## EQUATION 1
## Link function for mu1: probit
## Formula: agree ~ s(bonus, bs = "re") + age + prearn + benefit + gender +
##     ethnicity
##
## Parametric coefficients:
##                Estimate Std. Error z value Pr(>|z|)
## (Intercept) -3.937e+00  1.063e+00  -3.703 0.000213 ***
## age         -2.157e-03  2.417e-03  -0.893 0.372016
## prearn      -3.032e-05  1.035e-05  -2.929 0.003399 **
## benefit     -1.937e-03  5.090e-04  -3.806 0.000141 ***
## gender       1.493e-01  4.328e-02   3.449 0.000563 ***
## ethnicity    7.004e-02  4.869e-02   1.439 0.150258
## ---
## Signif. codes:  0 '***' 0.001 '**' 0.01 '*' 0.05 '.' 0.1 ' ' 1
##
## Approximate significance of smooth terms:
##            edf Ref.df Chi.sq  p-value
## s(bonus) 0.9516      1   19.7 5.86e-06 ***
## ---
## Signif. codes:  0 '***' 0.001 '**' 0.01 '*' 0.05 '.' 0.1 ' ' 1
##
##
## EQUATION 2
## Link function for mu2: probit
## Formula: status ~ agree * gender + s(age) + s(prearn) + benefit
##       + ethnicity
## Parametric coefficients:
##                Estimate Std. Error z value Pr(>|z|)
## (Intercept)  -0.4045767  0.0621760  -6.507 7.67e-11 ***
## agree         0.0894306  0.0620291   1.442 0.149372
## gender        0.1702680  0.0394460   4.316 1.59e-05 ***
## benefit      -0.0025938  0.0003999  -6.486 8.80e-11 ***
## ethnicity    -0.1404866  0.0363815  -3.861 0.000113 ***
## agree:gender -0.0498655  0.0667842  -0.747 0.455264
## ---
## Signif. codes:  0 '***' 0.001 '**' 0.01 '*' 0.05 '.' 0.1 ' ' 1
```

```
##
## Approximate significance of smooth terms:
##              edf Ref.df Chi.sq p-value
## s(age)     1.278  1.506  0.124 0.87409
## s(prearn) 2.597  3.309 12.811 0.00781 **
## ---
## Signif. codes:  0 '***' 0.001 '**' 0.01 '*' 0.05 '.' 0.1 ' ' 1
##
...
```

Males are significantly more likely to agree to participate in the experiment than females, reflecting gender-related differences in job-seeking behavior and responses to labor market policies. Moreover, individuals with higher earnings prior to unemployment may feel less financially constrained, resulting in a decreased probability of joining the program. Larger unemployment benefits also lower the likelihood of enrolling.

The effect of the instrumental variable and the associated interval are extracted as follows.

```
cb <- as.numeric(coef(out)["s(bonus).1"])
sb <- qnorm(0.975)*out$Vb["s(bonus).1","s(bonus).1"]
c(cb, cb - sb, cb + sb)
```

```
## [1] 4.685256 2.482623 6.887888
```

As expected, the presence of a **bonus** provides an incentive, making individuals more likely to agree to participate in the program.

In the reemployment equation, being Black and receiving higher unemployment benefits are associated with lower probabilities of reemployment, which may reflect systemic barriers that affect Black individuals in the labor market and the possibility that individuals receiving substantial benefits may feel less urgency to secure a job quickly. Conversely, as illustrated in Figure 12.1, pre-earnings have a notable impact on the reemployment likelihood, increasing it up to approximately $8,000. Beyond this point, the relationship appears to reverse, although the intervals are wide due to the sparsity of the data. Age does not appear to play a role here, possibly due to the balancing effects of age-related characteristics, such as experience and skills, across different age groups.

```
par(mfrow = c(1, 2))
plot(out, eq = 2, scale = 0, select = 1)
plot(out, eq = 2, scale = 0, select = 2)
```

Following Han and Vytlacil [2017], an additional recursive bivariate model is considered, where the margins are modeled using **probit** links and the copula is a 90° rotated Joe.

```
outJ90  <- gjrm(fl, data = hie, margins = c("probit", "probit"),
                copula = "J90", model = "B")
ATE(outJ90,  trt = "agree", int.var = c("agree:gender", 0))
```

```
##
## Average treatment effect with 95% interval:
##
## 0.0287 (-0.0075,0.0754)
```

```
ATE(outJ90, trt = "agree", int.var = c("agree:gender", 1))
```

```
##
## Average treatment effect with 95% interval:
##
## 0.0127 (-0.0201,0.0409)
```

The ATEs are consistent with previous results.

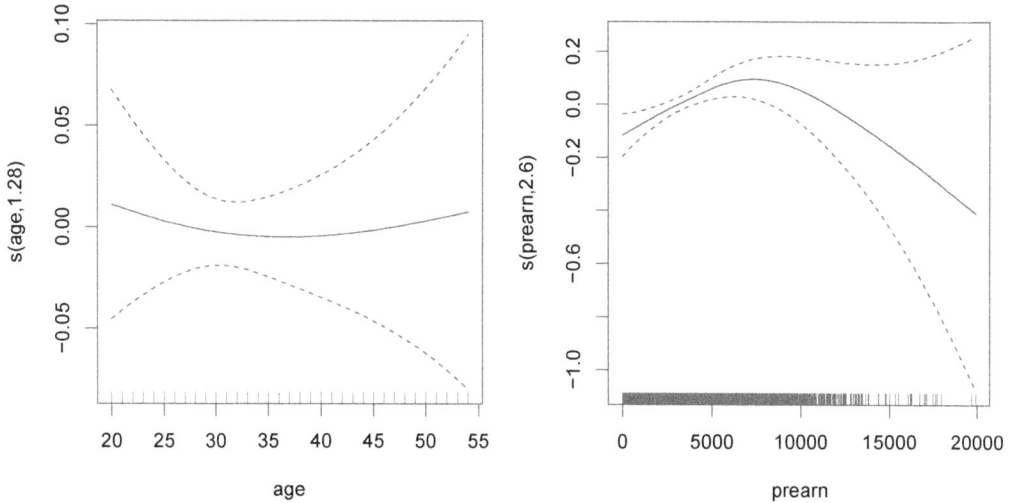

FIGURE 12.1 Estimated smooth effects (with associated 95% intervals) of `age` and `prearn` on the scale of the additive predictor of the reemployment equation, derived from a recursive bivariate probit model fitted to the `hie` data.

12.5   Trivariate extension

GJRM supports the specification of a trivariate binary additive regression model, as outlined in Section 5.5. This may be useful for estimating the effects of two endogenous binary treatments on a binary outcome. As an example, one might be interested in assessing how two different reemployment strategies affect the probability of securing a job, while accounting for the endogeneity of individual participation choices.

An illustration using simulated data is provided below.

```
data(dataDE)
```

```
eq1 <- y1 ~           x1 + x2 + x3 # first  endogenous variable
eq2 <- y2 ~           x1 + x2 + x4 # second endogenous variable
eq3 <- y3 ~ y1 + y2 + x1 + x2      # outcome
fl  <- list(eq1, eq2, eq3)
```

```
margs <- c("probit", "probit", "probit")
b      <- gjrm(fl, data = dataDE, margins = margs, model = "T")

conv.check(b)

##
## Maximum absolute gradient value: 3.214576e-09
## Observed information matrix is positive definite
ATE(b, eq = 3, trt = "y1")

##
## Average treatment effect with 95% interval:
##
## 0.3150 (0.0263,0.5383)
ATE(b, eq = 3, trt = "y2")

##
## Average treatment effect with 95% interval:
##
## -0.207 (-0.292,-0.149)
```

The ATEs are calculated by adapting equation (12.1) to this context.

13

Time-to-event outcome with binary treatment effect

This chapter explores a method for estimating the causal effect of a binary treatment on a survival outcome, in the presence of observed and unobserved confounders. This problem has been studied using various methods [Chernozhukov et al., 2015, Li et al., 2015, Martinussen et al., 2017, Sant'Anna, 2021, Beyhum et al., 2022]. The structural equation approach discussed here utilizes a bivariate Gaussian distribution to link a monotone transformation of the time-to-event and the propensity to be treated [Marra and Radice, 2025c].

The model is employed to reanalyze a dataset from the Illinois Reemployment Bonus Experiment, introduced in Chapter 12, to isolate the causal effect of a cash bonus on unemployment duration. The results show that the bonus significantly reduces the probability of remaining unemployed among women at different time points. If unobserved confounding is not addressed, the impact of the incentive is underestimated and deemed not significant.

13.1 Model

Consider a pair of random variables (Y_1, T_2), where Y_1 represents the binary treatment and T_2 denotes the time-to-event. The follow-up time is defined as $Y_2 = \min(T_2, C)$, where C is the right censoring time, independent of T_2. Next, assume that $Y_1 \sim \mathrm{Ber}(\mu_1)$ with $\mu_1 = \Phi\{\eta_{\mu_1}(\boldsymbol{x}_{\mu_1}; \boldsymbol{\beta}_{\mu_1})\}$, where $\boldsymbol{x}_{\mu_1} = (\boldsymbol{x}_o^\top, \boldsymbol{x}_{iv}^\top)^\top$ includes observed confounders and at least an instrumental variable satisfying the requirements detailed in Section 12.2, and $\boldsymbol{\beta}_{\mu_1} = (\boldsymbol{\beta}_{o\mu_1}^\top, \boldsymbol{\beta}_{iv}^\top)^\top$. For the outcome, $L(T_2) \sim \mathcal{N}(\eta_{\mu_2}(\boldsymbol{x}_{\mu_2}; \boldsymbol{\beta}_{\mu_2}), 1)$, where $L(\cdot)$ is an increasing monotonic transformation function (see Section 1.1.1), $\boldsymbol{x}_{\mu_2} = (\boldsymbol{x}_o^\top, y_1)^\top$ includes observed confounders and the treatment, and $\boldsymbol{\beta}_{\mu_2} = (\boldsymbol{\beta}_{o\mu_2}^\top, \beta_{tr})^\top$.

The survival transformation model can be expressed as

$$S(t_2) = \Phi\left\{-L(t_2) + \eta_{\mu_2}(\boldsymbol{x}_{\mu_2}; \boldsymbol{\beta}_{\mu_2})\right\} = \Phi\left\{-\eta_S(\boldsymbol{x}_S; \boldsymbol{\beta}_S)\right\},$$

where $S(t_2)$ is the survival function of T_2, $-L(t_2)$ is the baseline survival and $\eta_S(\boldsymbol{x}_S; \boldsymbol{\beta}_S)$ is an additive predictor depending on $\boldsymbol{x}_S = (t_2, \boldsymbol{x}_{\mu_2}^\top)^\top$ and parameter vector $\boldsymbol{\beta}_S$. The model specification is completed by coupling the CDF of Y_1 with $S(t_2)$ via a Gaussian copula.

13.2 Log-likelihood

For an observed sample $(y_{i2}, \boldsymbol{x}_i)_{i=1}^n$, where $\boldsymbol{x}_i$ is the union of $\boldsymbol{x}_{i\mu_1}$ and $\boldsymbol{x}_{i\mu_2}$, the log-likelihood of the mixed binary and time-to-event outcomes copula regression model is

DOI: 10.1201/9781003593195-13

$$\ell(\boldsymbol{\delta}) = \sum_{i=1}^{n} \Big[(1 - y_{i1})\, 1\{T_{i2} > C_i\} \log \{\Phi_2(-\eta_{\mu_{i1}}, -\eta_{S_i}; \theta)\}$$

$$+ y_{i1} 1\{T_{i2} > C_i\} \log \{\Phi(-\eta_{S_i}) - \Phi_2(-\eta_{\mu_{i1}}, -\eta_{S_i}; \theta)\}$$

$$+ (1 - y_{i1})\, 1\{T_{i2} \le C_i\} \log \left\{ -\frac{\partial \Phi_2(-\eta_{\mu_{i1}}, -\eta_{S_i}; \theta)}{\partial \Phi(-\eta_{S_i})} \frac{\partial \Phi(-\eta_{S_i})}{\partial \eta_{S_i}} \frac{\partial \eta_{S_i}}{\partial y_{i2}} \right\}$$

$$+ y_{i1} 1\{T_{i2} \le C_i\} \log \left\{ -\frac{\partial \Phi(-\eta_{S_i})}{\partial \eta_{S_i}} \frac{\partial \eta_{S_i}}{\partial y_{i2}} - \frac{\partial \Phi_2(-\eta_{\mu_{i1}}, -\eta_{S_i}; \theta)}{\partial \Phi(-\eta_{S_i})} \frac{\partial \Phi(-\eta_{S_i})}{\partial \eta_{S_i}} \frac{\partial \eta_{S_i}}{\partial y_{i2}} \right\} \Big] ,$$

where $\eta_{\mu_{i1}}$ and η_{S_i} are the shorthand notations for $\eta_{\mu_1}(\boldsymbol{x}_{\mu_1}; \boldsymbol{\beta}_{i\mu_1})$ and $\eta_S(\boldsymbol{x}_{iS}; \boldsymbol{\beta}_S)$, respectively, and $\boldsymbol{x}_{iS} = \left(y_{i2}, \boldsymbol{x}_{i\mu_2}^{\top}\right)^{\top}$. The term $\partial \eta_{S_i}/\partial y_{i2}$ is conveniently calculated by finite differencing (see Marra and Radice [2025c] for more details).

13.3   Survival average treatment effect

The estimator of the survival average treatment effect (SATE) at time t is defined as

$$\text{SATE}(t; \hat{\boldsymbol{\beta}}_S) = \frac{1}{n} \sum_{i=1}^{n} \left(\Phi\left[-\eta_S \left\{ \left(t, \boldsymbol{x}_{io}^{\top}, 1\right)^{\top}; \hat{\boldsymbol{\beta}}_S \right\} \right] - \Phi\left[-\eta_{Si} \left\{ \left(t, \boldsymbol{x}_{io}^{\top}, 0\right)^{\top}; \hat{\boldsymbol{\beta}}_S \right\} \right] \right).$$

Intervals are conveniently obtained through posterior simulation.

13.4   Model fitting

The dataset and problem description are discussed in Chapter 12, to which the reader is referred for details.

The equations for the treatment and time-to-event, `agree` and `unemp.dur`, are

```
library(GJRM); library(GJRM.data)
data(hie)

eq1 <- agree      ~ s(bonus, bs = "re") + age + prearn + benefit +
                    gender + ethnicity
eq2 <- unemp.dur ~ s(unemp.dur, bs = "mpi") + agree*gender + s(age) +
                    s(prearn) + benefit + ethnicity
fl  <- list(eq1, eq2)
```

This specification is the same as that adopted in Section 12.4, but `eq2` now includes a smooth term for the time variable, as required by the model.

```
out <- gjrm(fl, data = hie, margins = c("probit", "-probit"),
            cens2 = status, model = "B", uni.fit = TRUE)
```

```
conv.check(out)
```

```
##
## Maximum absolute gradient value: 0.02523672
## Observed information matrix is positive definite
summary(out, n.sim = 1000)

...
##
## theta = -0.0821(-0.159,-0.00502)
## n = 7734   total edf = 26.9
```

Convergence checks are adequate, and the estimated correlation parameter is negative and significant. This indicates that unobserved confounders increase both the likelihood of individuals joining the program and their probability of remaining unemployed. Failing to account for them will result in an underestimation of the impact of being part of the HIE group on the probability of staying unemployed.

The SATEs for weeks 1–25, in intervals of three weeks, by gender, derived from the joint and univariate models, are presented below.

```
t.grid <- seq(1, 25, by = 3)
SATE(out, trt = "agree", surv.t = t.grid, int.var = c("agree:gender", 0))
```

```
##
## Survival average treatment effects with 95% intervals:
##
##   surv.t    SATE    2.5%     97.5%
## 1      1 -0.0133 -0.0230 -0.00199
## 2      4 -0.0250 -0.0436 -0.00379
## 3      7 -0.0315 -0.0543 -0.00481
## 4     10 -0.0352 -0.0600 -0.00546
## 5     13 -0.0380 -0.0649 -0.00594
## 6     16 -0.0405 -0.0693 -0.00632
## 7     19 -0.0424 -0.0724 -0.00661
## 8     22 -0.0445 -0.0760 -0.00700
## 9     25 -0.0465 -0.0790 -0.00734
SATE(out, trt = "agree", surv.t = t.grid, int.var = c("agree:gender", 1))
```

```
##
## Survival average treatment effects with 95% intervals:
##
##   surv.t     SATE    2.5%    97.5%
## 1      1 -0.00354 -0.0133 0.00742
## 2      4 -0.00684 -0.0253 0.01461
## 3      7 -0.00867 -0.0323 0.01871
## 4     10 -0.00977 -0.0364 0.02107
## 5     13 -0.01059 -0.0395 0.02269
## 6     16 -0.01133 -0.0422 0.02407
## 7     19 -0.01189 -0.0443 0.02515
## 8     22 -0.01253 -0.0468 0.02667
## 9     25 -0.01314 -0.0488 0.02818
```

```
SATE(out, trt = "agree", joint = FALSE, surv.t = t.grid,
     int.var = c("agree:gender", 0))
```

```
##
## Survival average treatment effects with 95% intervals:
##
##    surv.t     SATE     2.5%    97.5%
## 1       1 -0.00585 -0.0166  0.00284
## 2       4 -0.01114 -0.0312  0.00548
## 3       7 -0.01403 -0.0390  0.00694
## 4      10 -0.01575 -0.0433  0.00785
## 5      13 -0.01702 -0.0466  0.00852
## 6      16 -0.01816 -0.0496  0.00911
## 7      19 -0.01901 -0.0517  0.00957
## 8      22 -0.02000 -0.0543  0.01010
## 9      25 -0.02090 -0.0566  0.01059
```

```
SATE(out, trt = "agree", joint = FALSE, surv.t = t.grid,
     int.var = c("agree:gender", 1))
```

```
##
## Survival average treatment effects with 95% intervals:
##
##    surv.t    SATE      2.5%   97.5%
## 1       1 0.00268 -0.00279  0.0102
## 2       4 0.00519 -0.00508  0.0197
## 3       7 0.00660 -0.00640  0.0252
## 4      10 0.00745 -0.00715  0.0284
## 5      13 0.00808 -0.00772  0.0308
## 6      16 0.00866 -0.00824  0.0329
## 7      19 0.00909 -0.00862  0.0345
## 8      22 0.00960 -0.00913  0.0364
## 9      25 0.01007 -0.00955  0.0384
```

The estimates from the joint model indicate that the cash bonus significantly reduces the probability of remaining unemployed for women. This is visually represented in Figure 13.1, which further shows that the survival function for the treatment group is consistently lower than that for the control group. Gender-specific differences in job-seeking behavior, such as motivation to find a job, may explain this result. Furthermore, women may face distinct challenges in the labor market, making the incentive particularly relevant for them. The R code used to produce Figure 13.1 is available on the authors' websites.

For interpretation, consider week 22. The probability of staying unemployed is 4.5 percentage points lower for women in the HIE group relative to the control group when accounting for unobserved confounding, compared to a non-statistically significant decrease of only two percentage points when neglecting it.

Further results are discussed below, focusing on the time-to-event equation as the covariate effects in the treatment equation are, as expected, virtually identical to those reported in Chapter 12.

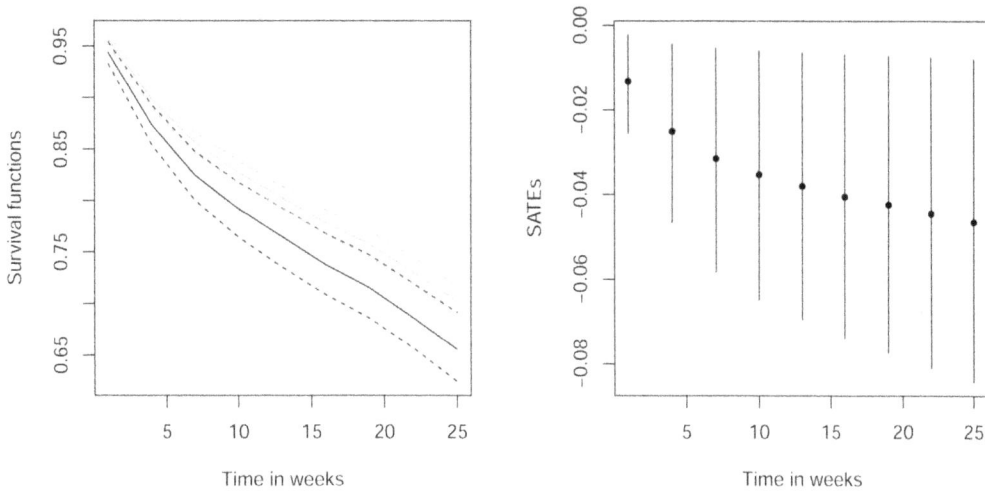

FIGURE 13.1 Estimated survival functions for the treatment and control groups (black and gray lines, respectively) and corresponding SATEs, with 95% intervals, for females, derived from a causal survival model fitted to the `hie` data.

```
summary(out)

...
##
## EQUATION 2
## Formula: unemp.dur ~ s(unemp.dur, bs = "mpi") + agree * gender + s(age) +
##      s(prearn) + benefit + ethnicity
##
## Parametric coefficients:
##                Estimate Std. Error z value Pr(>|z|)
## (Intercept)  -0.6235114  0.0602102 -10.356  < 2e-16 ***
## agree         0.1316949  0.0609509   2.161   0.0307 *
## gender        0.1721638  0.0381171   4.517 6.28e-06 ***
## benefit      -0.0025156  0.0003871  -6.498 8.13e-11 ***
## ethnicity    -0.2145266  0.0351837  -6.097 1.08e-09 ***
## agree:gender -0.0936499  0.0646614  -1.448   0.1475
## ---
## Signif. codes:  0 '***' 0.001 '**' 0.01 '*' 0.05 '.' 0.1 ' ' 1
##
## Approximate significance of smooth terms:
##                edf Ref.df    Chi.sq p-value
## s(unemp.dur) 8.584  8.886 13161.332  <2e-16 ***
## s(age)       2.016  2.532     4.489  0.1786
## s(prearn)    2.331  2.978     8.452  0.0339 *
## ---
## Signif. codes:  0 '***' 0.001 '**' 0.01 '*' 0.05 '.' 0.1 ' ' 1
##
...
```

Recall that a `-probit` link is employed to specify the time-to-event equation. This means that positive (negative) coefficients or upward (downward) trends in the estimated relationships correspond to shorter (longer) durations of unemployment. Being Black and receiving higher benefits are associated with longer durations of unemployment. As illustrated in Figure 13.2, pre-earnings significantly influence the duration of unemployment, reducing it up to around $8,000. Beyond this threshold, the relationship seems to reverse, although the intervals widen considerably due to the sparsity of the data. Age does not appear to be associated with the outcome, which may be due to the balancing effects of age-related factors. Lastly, consistent with the model design, the baseline smooth function for the duration variable shows a monotonically increasing trend, indicating that individuals generally experience shorter unemployment periods as time progresses.

```
par(mfrow = c(1, 3))
plot(out, eq = 2, scale = 0, select = 1)
plot(out, eq = 2, scale = 0, select = 2)
plot(out, eq = 2, scale = 0, select = 3, rug = TRUE, jit = TRUE)
```

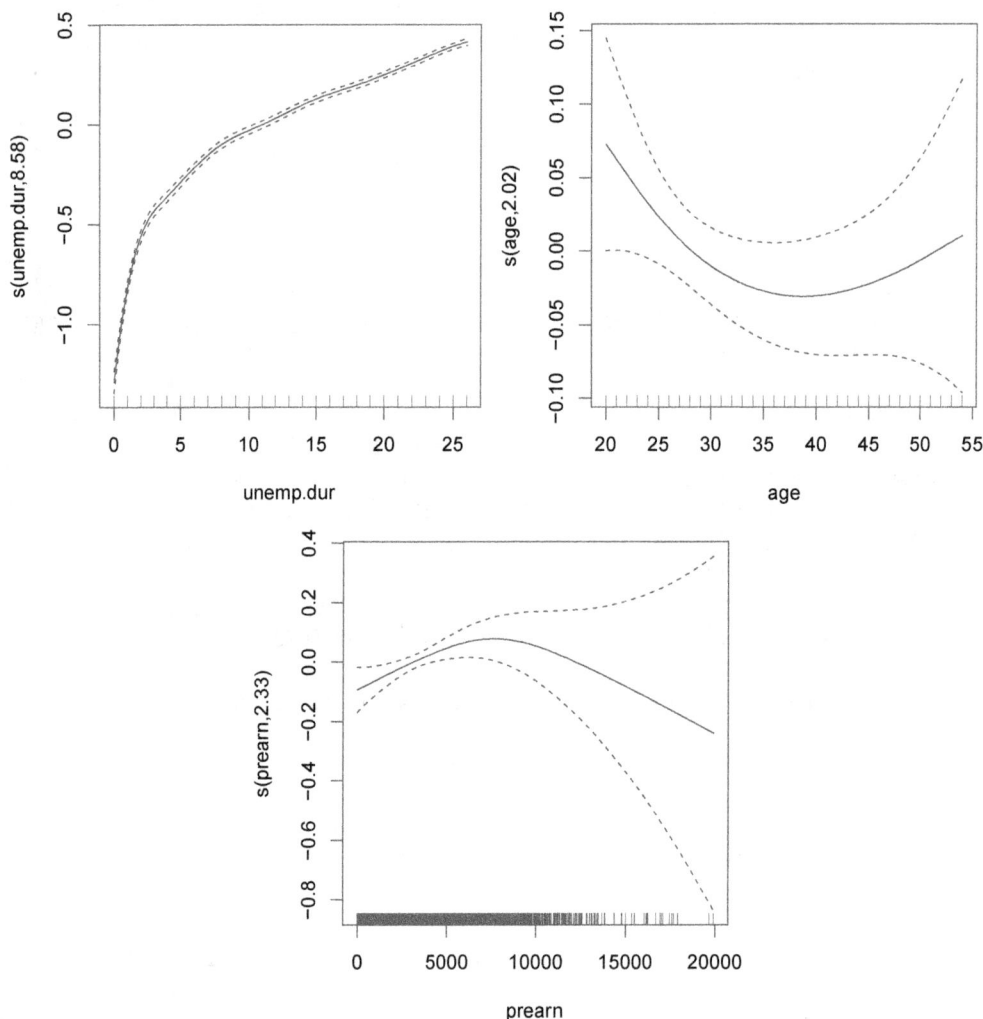

FIGURE 13.2 Estimated smooth effects (with associated 95% intervals) of `unemp.dur`, `age` and `prearn` on the scale of the additive predictor of the survival function of unemployment duration, derived from a causal survival model fitted to the `hie` data.

14

Binary outcome with missingness not at random

Nonrandom sample selection occurs when the likelihood of an outcome being missing (or observed) depends on its value. Addressing this issue requires controlling for unobserved confounders, as failing to account for them can lead to inconsistent parameter estimates. Simultaneous modeling of the outcome and missing mechanism, using the sample selection approach by Marra et al. [2017], addresses this problem in the case of a binary response. For an overview of models dealing with missingness not at random, see Fitzmaurice et al. [2008, Chapter 18].

The potential of the sample selection approach is illustrated using synthetic HIV prevalence data from Zambia. This example highlights the challenges associated with an outcome that has missing values not occurring at random, as participation in HIV testing can be influenced by the HIV status of individuals.

14.1 HIV population study

Understanding HIV prevalence is essential for informing public health policy, assessing the overall health of a population and evaluating the effectiveness of interventions. However, obtaining accurate prevalence estimates can be challenging, as they often rely on data from household surveys where participation in testing may be low, especially among HIV-positive individuals who fear disclosure. This selective participation may lead to underestimated figures for HIV prevalence if the analysis focuses solely on the observed outcome (HIV status) without accounting for the selection process (consent to test). In such a case, unobserved confounding plays a crucial role as it influences both an individual's likelihood of consenting to HIV testing and their HIV status. For example, HIV-positive individuals may be less inclined to participate in the survey due to fears of stigma, resulting in an underrepresentation of HIV-positive cases. The framework discussed here addresses this challenge by simultaneously modeling HIV status and consent to test.

The approach is applied to a case study estimating HIV prevalence among Zambian men, using synthetic data with a sample size of 6,416 that replicates the structure and statistical properties of the 2007 Demographic and Health Surveys.

14.2 Model

Consider a pair of binary random variables (Y_1, Y_2), where Y_1 represents the selection mechanism, Y_2 is the outcome (observed only if $Y_1 = 1$), and Y_1 and Y_2 are assumed to be associated through unobserved confounders.

DOI: 10.1201/9781003593195-14

Y_1 and Y_2 follow Bernoulli distributions with parameters $g_{\mu_1}(\mu_1) = \eta_{\mu_1}(\boldsymbol{x}_{\mu_1}; \boldsymbol{\beta}_{\mu_1})$ and $g_{\mu_2}(\mu_2) = \eta_{\mu_2}(\boldsymbol{x}_{\mu_2}; \boldsymbol{\beta}_{\mu_2})$, where $\boldsymbol{x}_{\mu_1} = (\boldsymbol{x}_o^\top, \boldsymbol{x}_{iv}^\top)^\top$ contains observed confounders and at least an instrumental variable satisfying the requirements detailed in Section 12.2, $\boldsymbol{x}_{\mu_2}$ includes observed confounders only, and $\boldsymbol{\beta}_{\mu_1} = (\boldsymbol{\beta}_{o\mu_1}^\top, \boldsymbol{\beta}_{iv}^\top)^\top$. The model specification is completed by joining the CDFs of Y_1 and Y_2 via a copula function, as in equation (5.1), with dependence parameter $g_\theta(\theta) = \eta_\theta(\boldsymbol{x}_\theta; \boldsymbol{\beta}_\theta)$. For identification, the copula function and its margins are classically specified as Gaussian and probit. However, by analogy with the recursive bivariate probit model discussed in Chapter 12, non-Gaussian distributions may also be considered.

In this framework, there are three possible events. The first is $Y_1 = 0$, which occurs with probability $\mathbb{P}(Y_1 = 0) = F_1(0; \mu_1)$. The second is $Y_1 = 1$ and $Y_2 = 1$, with joint probability $\mathbb{P}(Y_1 = 1, Y_2 = 1) = C(F_1(1; \mu_1), F_2(1; \mu_2); \theta)$. Finally, the third event is $Y_1 = 1$ and $Y_2 = 0$, with probability $\mathbb{P}(Y_1 = 1, Y_2 = 0) = \mathbb{P}(Y_1 = 1) - \mathbb{P}(Y_1 = 1, Y_2 = 1)$.

14.3   Log-likelihood

For an observed sample $(y_{i1}, y_{i2}, \boldsymbol{x}_i)_{i=1}^n$, where the covariate vector $\boldsymbol{x}_i$ is the union of $\boldsymbol{x}_{i\mu_1}$, $\boldsymbol{x}_{i\mu_2}$ and $\boldsymbol{x}_{i\theta}$, the log-likelihood of the binary sample selection model is

$$
\begin{aligned}
\ell(\boldsymbol{\beta}) = \sum_{i=1}^n & [y_{i1} y_{i2} \log C(F_1(1; \mu_{i1}), F_2(1; \mu_{i2}); \theta_i) + y_{i1}(1 - y_{i2}) \log \{F_1(1; \mu_{i1}) \\
& - C(F_1(1; \mu_{i1}), F_2(1; \mu_{i2}); \theta_i)\} + (1 - y_{i1}) \log F_1(0; \mu_{i1})]
\end{aligned}
$$

where $\boldsymbol{\beta} = (\boldsymbol{\beta}_{\mu_1}^\top, \boldsymbol{\beta}_{\mu_2}^\top, \boldsymbol{\beta}_\theta^\top)^\top$ is the overall regression coefficient vector.

14.4   Prevalence

In selection models, a measure of interest is prevalence, which can be estimated using

$$
\sum_{i=1}^n w_i F_2(1; \hat{\mu}_{i2}) / \sum_{i=1}^n w_i, \tag{14.1}
$$

where w_i represents the ith survey weight. Intervals are conveniently obtained through posterior simulation.

14.5   Model fitting

The selection and outcome equations are based on the same set of observed confounders. However, the selection equation also includes the instrumental variable `interviewerID`. The identity of the interviewer who contacts the respondent to seek consent for an HIV test is often recorded in survey data as an anonymized code. Interviewers in these surveys are frequently matched to participants based on group-level characteristics (e.g., language) rather than the characteristics of the respondents themselves. Therefore, interviewer identity is plausibly exogenous and is not expected to be associated with the HIV status of survey respondents [Marra et al., 2017].

Some interviewers either consistently succeed or fail to obtain consent for testing from all of their interviewees. This lack of within-interviewer variation in participation can lead to estimation issues. To address this problem, the approach discussed in Section 1.2.1 is employed.

```
library(GJRM); library(GJRM.data)
data(hiv)

sel.eq <- consent ~ age + education + wealth + region + marital + std +
                    agehadsex + highhiv + partner + condom + aidscare +
                    knowsdiedofaids + evertestedHIV + smoke + religion +
                    ethnicity + language + s(interviewerID, bs = "re")
out.eq <- status ~ age + education + wealth + region + marital + std +
                   agehadsex + highhiv + partner + condom + aidscare +
                   knowsdiedofaids + evertestedHIV + smoke + religion +
                   ethnicity + language
fl <- list(sel.eq, out.eq)

out <- gjrm(fl, data = hiv, margins = c("probit", "probit"), model = "BSS")
conv.check(out)
```

```
##
## Maximum absolute gradient value: 0.0003156494
## Observed information matrix is positive definite
```

Convergence checks are adequate, while the prevalences derived from both the joint and univariate models are presented next.

```
prev(out, sw = hiv$sw)
```

```
##
## Prevalence with 95% interval:
##
## 0.239 (0.201,0.294)
```

```
prev(out, sw = hiv$sw, joint = FALSE)
```

```
##
## Prevalence with 95% interval:
##
## 0.122 (0.117,0.132)
```

The estimate that accounts for nonrandom sample selection is twice as high as the one from the univariate model which ignores it. This finding aligns with the preconception that individuals who do not consent to testing are more likely to be HIV positive compared to those who do.

```
summary(out, n.sim = 1000)

...
##
## theta = -0.86(-0.95,-0.637)
...
```

The negative correlation supports this assumption, suggesting that individuals who participate in testing systematically differ in HIV status from those who do not, reflecting the bias introduced by the selection process.

Prevalence estimates can also be displayed by region using the information from `hiv.polys`, which contains a list of polygon vertices defining the boundaries of the Zambian regions. An example is reported here.

```
data(hiv.polys)
lr <- length(hiv.polys); prevBYreg <- matrix(NA, lr, 2)

for(i in 1:lr) {
  sws <- hiv$sw; sws[hiv$region != i] <- 0
  prevBYreg[i, 1] <- prev(out, sw = sws)$prev
  prevBYreg[i, 2] <- prev(out, sw = sws, joint = FALSE)$prev
}

par(mfrow = c(1, 2)); zr <- range(prevBYreg)
polys.map(hiv.polys, prevBYreg[, 1], zlim = zr)
polys.map(hiv.polys, prevBYreg[, 2], zlim = zr)
```

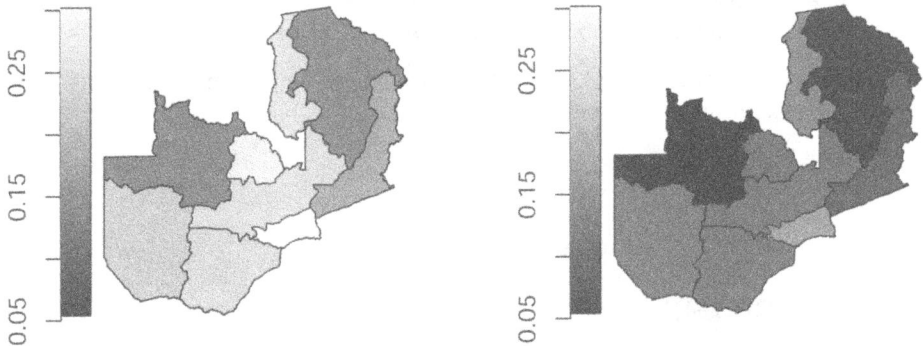

FIGURE 14.1 Regional HIV prevalence estimates for Zambia, derived from sample selection (left) and univariate probit (right) models fitted to the `hiv` data.

As illustrated in Figure 14.1, the sample selection estimates range from 15% in Northwestern Zambia to 30% in Lusaka, while those neglecting selective sampling range from 5% to 18%. The variation observed among regions can be attributed to demographic and socioeconomic influences.

Several variables are associated with both the propensity to consent to HIV testing and the likelihood of being HIV positive. The results are not displayed here due to the lengthy nature of the R output, but they can be visualized using `summary(out)`. These relationships are commented below.

Older individuals and those with higher education levels are more likely to undergo testing, possibly due to their greater awareness of HIV and its implications. Individuals engaging in high-risk sexual practices have a greater tendency to seek testing, presumably driven by a desire to stay informed. Similarly, having cared for an HIV-infected relative or knowing someone who has died as a result of HIV significantly increases the likelihood of consenting to testing. Ethnicity also plays a role, with members of the Tumbuka ethnic group showing a significantly higher propensity for testing compared to individuals from the Bemba group, possibly due to cultural shifts or heightened HIV awareness within the Tumbuka population.

Elderly individuals are at greater risk of testing positive, which may reflect longer exposure to risk factors over time. The positive relationship between wealth and HIV status could be attributed to wealthier individuals having greater mobility or engaging in riskier sexual activities, both of which increase their exposure to HIV. This suggests that in certain contexts, social and behavioral variables may outweigh the protective benefits of wealth. Being currently or formerly married is linked with a higher likelihood of being HIV positive compared to those who have never been married, possibly due to shared sexual networks among couples. A history of sexually transmitted diseases also significantly increases the risk of being HIV positive, reinforcing the established link between coinfections and elevated HIV risk.

Based on the arguments by Han and Vytlacil [2017] for recursive bivariate binary models, a 270° rotated Clayton sample selection model with `logit` margins is also fitted.

```
out2 <- gjrm(fl, data = hiv, margins = c("logit", "logit"), copula = "C270",
             model = "BSS")
prev(out2, sw = hiv$sw)


##
## Prevalence with 95% interval:
##
## 0.233 (0.203,0.278)
prev(out2, sw = hiv$sw, joint = FALSE)


##
## Prevalence with 95% interval:
##
## 0.122 (0.116,0.132)
```

The estimates are virtually identical to those previously reported.

To further demonstrate the potential of the framework, a more complex specification is explored, where the nonlinear effects of `age`, `education` and `wealth` are accounted for, and Gaussian Markov random field smooths are utilized to model the effects of `region` on all the distributional parameters.

```
xt <- list(polys = hiv.polys)

sel.eq <- consent ~ s(region, bs = "mrf", xt = xt) + s(age) + s(education) +
                    s(wealth) + marital + std + agehadsex + highhiv +
                    partner + condom + aidscare + knowsdiedofaids +
                    evertestedHIV + smoke + religion + ethnicity +
                    language + s(interviewerID, bs = "re")
```

```
out.eq <- status    ~ s(region, bs = "mrf", xt = xt) + s(age) + s(education) +
                      s(wealth) + marital + std + agehadsex + highhiv +
                      partner + condom + aidscare + knowsdiedofaids +
                      evertestedHIV + smoke + religion + ethnicity + language
theta.eq <-         ~ s(region, bs = "mrf", xt = xt)


fl <- list(sel.eq, out.eq, theta.eq)

out3 <- gjrm(fl, data = hiv, margins = c("probit", "probit"), model = "BSS")
prev(out3, sw = hiv$sw)

##
## Prevalence with 95% interval:
##
## 0.224 (0.196,0.272)
```

Although this model specification does not significantly affect the overall prevalence, it offers additional insights. For example, Figure 14.2 shows that individuals in the northern regions of Zambia are more likely to consent to HIV testing, which may reflect greater awareness driven by effective public health campaigns and strong community support. It also shows that the likelihood of consenting to HIV testing increases with education up to approximately 11 years, after which it declines, although the wide intervals beyond this point make any conclusions uncertain. Moreover, the likelihood of being HIV-positive increases with wealth up to a certain threshold, after which it stabilizes, showing no further effect. Lastly, there is evidence of a heterogeneous selection process across regions, with unobserved confounders influencing consent to testing and HIV status to varying degrees, possibly depending on local cultural and social conditions.

```
par(mfrow = c(2, 2))
plot(out3, eq = 1, scheme = 1, select = 1)
plot(out3, eq = 1, scheme = 1, select = 3, scale = 0,
     rug = TRUE, jit = TRUE)
plot(out3, eq = 2, scheme = 1, select = 4, scale = 0)
plot(out3, eq = 3, scheme = 1)
```

14.6   Trivariate extension

GJRM supports the specification of a trivariate binary double sample selection model, which can be considered a special case of the trivariate model discussed in Section 5.5. An example might involve a scenario where individuals are first contacted to participate in a survey, with some choosing not to respond. Among those who do respond, they then decide whether to consent to be part of the study.

Consider three binary random variables (Y_1, Y_2, Y_3), where Y_1 (respond to contact) and Y_2 (consent to test) represent the two selection mechanisms determining whether the outcome Y_3 is observed. The possible events are $Y_1 = 0$ (implying that Y_2 and Y_3 are missing); $Y_1 = 1$ and $Y_2 = 0$ (implying Y_3 is missing); $Y_1 = 1$, $Y_2 = 1$ and $Y_3 = 0$; $Y_1 = 1$, $Y_2 = 1$ and $Y_3 = 1$. Using the notation from Section 5.5, for an observed sample $(y_{i1}, y_{i2}, y_{i3}, \boldsymbol{x}_i)_{i=1}^n$, where the covariate vector $\boldsymbol{x}_i$ is the union of $\boldsymbol{x}_{i\mu_1}$, $\boldsymbol{x}_{i\mu_2}$ and $\boldsymbol{x}_{i\mu_3}$, the log-likelihood function of the

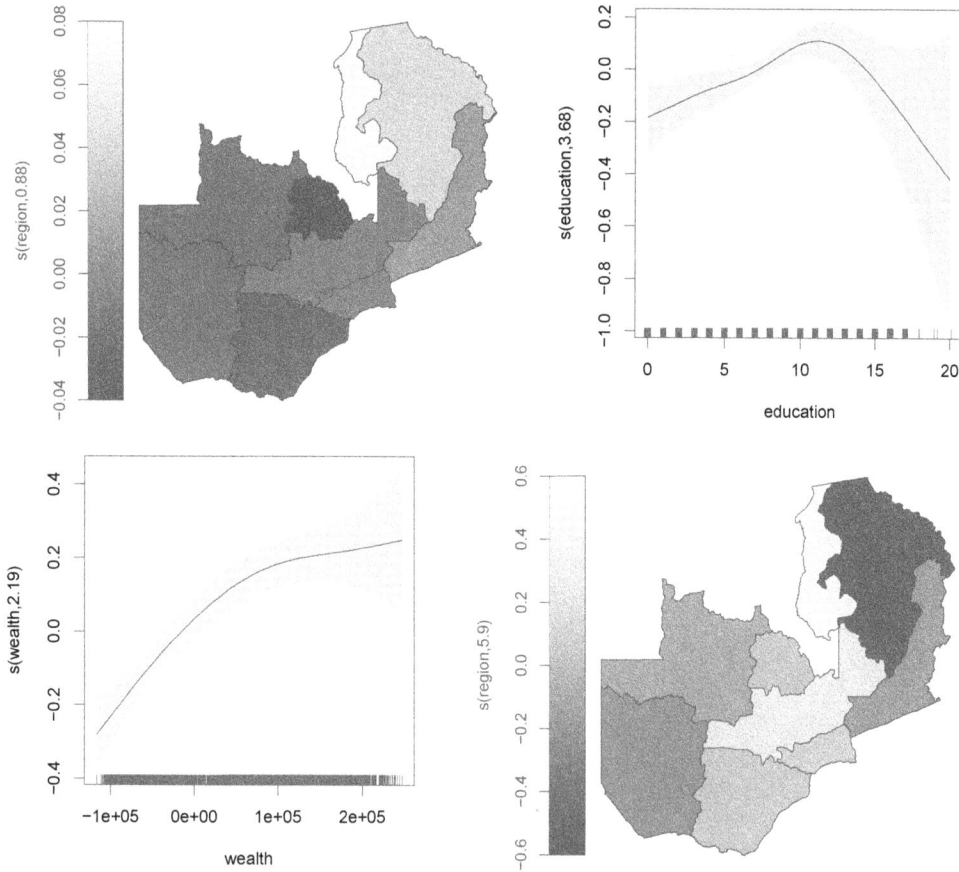

FIGURE 14.2 Estimated effects of `region` and `education` on the scale of the additive predictor of μ_1 (top plots), of `wealth` on the scale of the additive predictor of μ_2 (bottom left), and of `region` on the scale of the additive predictor of θ (bottom right), derived from a sample selection probit model fitted to the `hiv` data.

double sample selection model is

$$\ell(\boldsymbol{\beta}) = \sum_{i=1}^{n} \{(1 - y_{i1}) \log(1 - p_{i1}) + y_{i1}(1 - y_{i2}) \log(p_{i1} - p_{i12}) $$
$$+ y_{i1} y_{i2}(1 - y_{i3}) \log(p_{i12} - p_{i123}) + y_{i1} y_{i2} y_{i3} \log(p_{i123})\}$$

In this case, `GJRM` does not currently allow the dependence parameters to be specified as functions of covariate effects.

The model is illustrated below with simulated data.

```
data(dataDSS)
```

```
eq1 <- y1 ~ x1 + x2 + x3    # first selection
eq2 <- y2 ~ x1 + x2 + x4    # second selection
eq3 <- y3 ~ x1 + x2         # outcome variable
fl  <- list(eq1, eq2, eq3)
```

```
margs <- c("probit", "probit", "probit")
outt  <- gjrm(f1, data = dataDSS, margins = margs, model = "TSS")
conv.check(outt)
```

```
##
## Maximum absolute gradient value: 3.254169e-11
## Observed information matrix is positive definite
```

The mean of the fully observed outcome y3.o is

```
mean(dataDSS$y3.o)
```

```
## [1] 0.5674
```

The prevalences from the joint and univariate models are calculated using (14.1), where $F_2(1; \hat{\mu}_{i2})$ is replaced with $F_3(1; \hat{\mu}_{i3})$.

```
prev(outt)
```

```
##
## Prevalence with 95% interval:
##
## 0.592 (0.388,0.795)
```

```
prev(outt, joint = FALSE)
```

```
##
## Prevalence with 95% interval:
##
## 0.872 (0.851,0.886)
```

The estimate from the double sample selection model is close to the mean of y3.o, while the one that ignores the missing mechanism deviates significantly from it.

GJRM supports the specification of a trivariate binary model that accounts for endogeneity and nonrandom sample selection through the option model = "TESS". This approach integrates the methodologies and specifications outlined in this section and in Sections 5.5 and 12.5. Consider, for example, a study where individuals are initially asked whether they consent to receive a vaccine (Y_1). Their decisions may be influenced by unobserved confounders, such as personal beliefs and perceived risks, which are reflected in the selection process. In the second stage, those who agree to vaccination can choose between vaccine 1 and vaccine 2 (Y_2), allowing for the evaluation of the effect of Y_2 on a health outcome (Y_3), such as hospitalization (yes/no), adverse reaction (yes/no) or infection status (infected/not infected). The choice of vaccine may be influenced by past experiences and current health conditions, making it potentially endogenous.

References

J. M. Abowd and H. S. Farber. Job queues and the union status of workers. *Industrial and Labor Relations Review*, 35(3):354–367, 1982.

H. Akaike. Information theory and an extension of the maximum likelihood principle. In *Selected Papers of Hirotugu Akaike*, pages 199–213. Springer, 1998.

AREDS Group. The age-related eye disease study (areds): Design implications. *AREDS report no. 1. Controlled Clinical Trials*, 20(6):573–600, 1999.

N. H. Augustin, E. A. Sauleau, and S. N. Wood. On quantile quantile plots for generalized linear models. *Computational Statistics & Data Analysis*, 56(8):2404–2409, 2012.

N. Azadeh-Fard, N. Ghaffarzadegan, and J. A. Camelio. Can a patient's in-hospital length of stay and mortality be explained by early-risk assessments? *PLoS One*, 11(9):1–9, 2016.

J. Beyhum, J.-P. Florens, and I. Van Keilegom. Nonparametric instrumental regression with right censored duration outcomes. *Journal of Business & Economic Statistics*, 40(3): 1034–1045, 2022.

M. I. Bhatti and H. Q. Do. Recent development in copula and its applications to the energy, forestry and environmental sciences. *International Journal of Hydrogen Energy*, 44(36): 19453–19473, 2019.

M. J. Bhuyan, M. A. Islam, and M. S. Rahman. A bivariate Bernoulli model for analyzing malnutrition. *Health Services and Outcomes Research Methodology*, 18:109–127, 2018.

G. Bijwaard and G. Ridder. Correcting for selective compliance in a re-employment bonus experiment. *Journal of Econometrics*, 125(1–2):77–111, 2005.

B. F. Braumoeller, G. Marra, R. Radice, and A. Bradshaw. Flexible causal inference for political science. *Political Analysis*, 26(1):54–71, 2018.

D. Card and L. Giuliano. Peer effects and multiple equilibria in the risky behavior of friends. *The Review of Economics and Statistics*, 95(4):1130–1149, 2013.

J. F. Carriere. Bivariate survival models for coupled lives. *Scandinavian Actuarial Journal*, 2000(1):17–32, 2000.

P. J. Catalano and L. M. Ryan. Bivariate latent variable models for clustered discrete and continuous outcomes. *Journal of the American Statistical Association*, 87(419):651–658, 1992.

S. Chakraborty, M. Ghosh, T. Maiti, and A. Tewari. Bayesian neural networks for bivariate binary data: An application to prostate cancer study. *Statistics in Medicine*, 24(23): 3645–3662, 2005.

S. C. Cheng, L. J. Wei, and Z. Ying. Analysis of transformation models with censored data. *Biometrika*, 82(4):835–845, 1995.

V. Chernozhukov, I. Fernández-Val, and A. E. Kowalski. Quantile regression with censoring and endogeneity. *Journal of Econometrics*, 186(1):201–221, 2015.

U. Cherubini, E. Luciano, and W. Vecchiato. *Copula Methods in Finance*. John Wiley & Sons, 2004.

K. A. Clarke. A simple distribution-free test for nonnested model selection. *Political Analysis*, 15:347–363, 2007.

P. S. Clarke and F. Windmeijer. Instrumental variable estimators for binary outcomes. *Journal of the American Statistical Association*, 107(500):1638–1652, 2012.

C. Czado. *Analyzing Dependent Data with Vine Copulas: A Practical Guide with R*. Springer, 2019.

P. J. Danaher and M. S. Smith. Modeling multivariate distributions using copulas: Applications in marketing. *Marketing Science*, 30(1):4–21, 2011.

W. L. de Oliveira, C. A. Ribeiro Diniz, and M. Durbán. A class of bivariate regression models for discrete and/or continuous responses. *Communications in Statistics – Simulation and Computation*, 48(8):2359–2383, 2019.

M. Delporte, G. Molenberghs, S. Fieuws, and G. Verbeke. A joint normal-ordinal (probit) model for ordinal and continuous longitudinal data. *Biostatistics*, 26: kxae014, 2024.

K. A. Doksum and M. Gasko. On a correspondence between models in binary regression analysis and in survival analysis. *International Statistical Review*, 58(3):243–252, 1990.

F. Donat and G. Marra. Simultaneous equation penalized likelihood estimation of vehicle accident injury severity. *Journal of the Royal Statistical Society Series C*, 67(4):979–1001, 2018.

P. K. Dunn and G. K. Smyth. Randomized quantile residuals. *Journal of Computational and Graphical Statistics*, 5(3):236–244, 1996.

P. K. Dunn and G. K. Smyth. Series evaluation of Tweedie exponential dispersion model densities. *Statistics and Computing*, 15:267–280, 2005.

S. K. Eden, C. Li, and B. E. Shepherd. Nonparametric estimation of Spearman's rank correlation with bivariate survival data. *Biometrics*, 78(2):421–434, 2022.

J. Espasandín-Domínguez, C. Cadarso-Suárez, T. Kneib, G. Marra, N. Klein, R. Radice, O. Lado-Baleato, A. González Quintela, and F. Gude. Assessing the relationship between markers of glycemic control through flexible copula regression models. *Statistics in Medicine*, 38(27):5161–5181, 2019.

J. D. Fearon and D. D. Laitin. Ethnicity, insurgency, and civil war. *American Political Science Review*, 97(1):75–90, 2003.

P. Filippou, G. Marra, and R. Radice. Penalized likelihood estimation of a trivariate additive probit model. *Biostatistics*, 18(3):569–585, 2017.

P. Filippou, T. Kneib, G. Marra, and R. Radice. A trivariate additive regression model with arbitrary link functions and varying correlation matrix. *Journal of Statistical Planning and Inference*, 199:236–248, 2019.

G. Fitzmaurice, M. Davidian, G. Verbeke, and G. Molenberghs. *Longitudinal Data Analysis*. CRC Press, 2008.

M. G. Fitzmaurice and N. M. Laird. Regression models for a bivariate discrete and continuous outcome with clustering. *Journal of the American Statistical Association*, 90(431):845–852, 1995.

S. D. Foster and M. V. Bravington. A Poisson-Gamma model for analysis of ecological non-negative continuous data. *Environmental & Ecological Statistics*, 20(4):533–552, 2013.

D. A. Freedman. *Statistical Models and Causal Inference: A Dialogue with the Social Sciences*. Cambridge University Press, 2009.

E. W. Frees and E. A. Valdez. Understanding relationships using copulas. *North American Actuarial Journal*, 22(1):1–25, 1998.

E. W. Frees and P. Wang. Credibility using copulas. *North American Actuarial Journal*, 9 (2):31–48, 2005.

S. Gurmu and J. Elder. Generalized bivariate count data regression models. *Economics Letters*, 68(1):31–36, 2000.

S. Gurmu and J. Elder. Flexible bivariate count data regression models. *Journal of Business & Economic Statistics*, 30(2):265–274, 2012.

S. Han and E. J. Vytlacil. Identification in a generalization of bivariate probit models with dummy endogenous regressors. *Journal of Econometrics*, 199(1):63–73, 2017.

T. S. Han, P. Murray, J. Robin, P. Wilkinson, D. Fluck, and C. H. Fry. Evaluation of the association of length of stay in hospital and outcomes. *International Society for Quality in Health Care*, 34(2):1–9, 2022.

K. Hashizume, J. Tshuchida, and T. Sozu. Flexible use of copula-type model for dose-finding in drug combination clinical trial. *Biometrics*, 78(4):1651–1661, 2022.

J. Helliwell, R. Layard, and J. Sachs. World happiness report 2019. Technical report. Sustainable Development Solutions Network, 2019.

M. Hohberg, F. Donat, G. Marra, and T. Kneib. Beyond unidimensional poverty analysis using distributional copula models for mixed ordered-continuous outcomes. *Journal of the Royal Statistical Society Series C*, 70(5):1365–1390, 2021.

N. J. Horton and G. M. Fitzmaurice. Maximum likelihood estimation of bivariate logistic models for incomplete responses with indicators of ignorable and non-ignorable missingness. *Journal of the Royal Statistical Society Series C*, 51(3):281–295, 2002.

K. Imai, Z. Jiang, D. J. Greiner, R. Halen, and S. Shin. Experimental evaluation of algorithm-assisted human decision-making: Application to pretrial public safety assessment. *Journal of the Royal Statistical Society Series A*, 186(2):167–189, 2023.

A. Ivanova, G. Molenberghs, and G. Verbeke. Mixed models approaches for joint modeling of different types of responses. *Journal of Biopharmaceutical Statistics*, 26(4):601–618, 2016.

H. Joe. *Dependence Modeling with Copulas*. Chapman & Hall/CRC, 2014.

B. Jørgensen and M. C. Paes De Souza. Fitting Tweedie's compound Poisson model to insurance claims data. *Scandinavian Actuarial Journal*, 1994(1):69–93, 1994.

W. S. Kendall. Scale invariant correlations between genes and SNPs on human chromosome 1 reveal potential evolutionary mechanisms. *Journal of Theoretical Biology*, 245(2):329–340, 2007.

N. Klein, T. Kneib, G. Marra, R. Radice, S. Rokicki, and M. E. McGovern. Mixed binary-continuous copula regression models with application to adverse birth outcomes. *Statistics in Medicine*, 38(3):413–436, 2019.

M. T. Lee and G. A. Whitmore. Stochastic processes directed by randomized time. *Journal of Applied Probability*, 30(2):302–314, 1993.

J. Li, J. Fine, and A. Brookhart. Instrumental variable additive hazards models. *Biometrics*, 71(1):122–130, 2015.

H. F. Lingsma, A. Bottle, S. Middleton, J. Kievit, E. W. Steyerberg, and P. J. Marang van de Mheen. Evaluation of hospital outcomes: The relation between length-of-stay, readmission, and mortality in a large international administrative database. *BMC Health Services Research*, 18(116), 2018.

Y. Lu. Flexible (panel) regression models for bivariate count–continuous data with an insurance application. *Journal of the Royal Statistical Society Series A*, 182(4):1503–1521, 2019.

Z. Ma, T. E. Hanson, and Y. Y. Ho. Application of bivariate negative binomial regression model in analysing insurance count data. *Annals of Actuarial Science*, 11(2):390–411, 2017.

Z. Ma, T. E. Hanson, and Y. Y. Ho. Flexible bivariate correlated count data regression. *Statistics in Medicine*, 39(25):3476–3490, 2020.

G. Marra and R. Radice. Estimation of a semiparametric recursive bivariate probit model in the presence of endogeneity. *Canadian Journal of Statistics*, 39(2):259–279, 2011.

G. Marra and R. Radice. A penalized likelihood estimation approach to semiparametric sample selection binary response modeling. *Electronic Journal of Statistics*, 7:1432–1455, 2013a.

G. Marra and R. Radice. Estimation of a regression spline sample selection model. *Computational Statistics & Data Analysis*, 61:158–173, 2013b.

G. Marra and R. Radice. Bivariate copula additive models for location, scale and shape. *Computational Statistics & Data Analysis*, 112:99–113, 2017.

G. Marra and R. Radice. Copula link-based additive models for right-censored event time data. *Journal of the American Statistical Association*, 115(530):886–895, 2020.

G. Marra and R. Radice. GJRM: Generalized joint regression modelling. 0.2-6.8, 2025a. URL https://CRAN.R-project.org/package=GJRM.

G. Marra and R. Radice. Modeling physician visit frequency and costs using a copula additive distributional regression approach. *Submitted*, 2025b.

G. Marra and R. Radice. Estimating the impact of screening on lung cancer diagnosis timing using a semiparametric transformation survival model. *Submitted*, 2025c.

G. Marra, R. Radice, T. Bärnighausen, S. N. Wood, and M. E. McGovern. A simultaneous equation approach to estimating HIV prevalence with nonignorable missing responses. *Journal of the American Statistical Association*, 112(518):484–496, 2017.

G. Marra, M. Fasiolo, R. Radice, and R. Winkelmann. A flexible copula regression model with Bernoulli and Tweedie margins for estimating the effect of spending on mental health. *Health Economics*, 32(6):1305–1322, 2023.

T. Martinussen, Ditte D. Nørbo Sørensen, and S. Vansteelandt. Instrumental variables estimation under a structural Cox model. *Biostatistics*, 20(1):65–79, 2017.

C. McCulloch. Joint modelling of mixed outcome types using latent variables. *Statistical Methods in Medical Research*, 17(1):53–73, 2008.

M. E. McGovern, T. Bärnighausen, G. Marra, and R. Radice. On the assumption of bivariate normality in selection models. *Epidemiology*, 26(2):229–237, 2015.

J. S. Najita, Y. Li, and P. J. Catalano. A novel application of a bivariate regression model for binary and continuous outcomes to studies of fetal toxicity. *Journal of the Royal Statistical Society Series C*, 58(4):555–573, 2009.

B. Neelon, R. Anthopolos, and M. L. Miranda. A spatial bivariate probit model for correlated binary data with application to adverse birth outcomes. *Statistical Methods in Medical Research*, 23(2):119–133, 2014.

R. B. Nelsen. *An Introduction to Copulas*. Springer Series in Statistics, 2006.

M. D. Nieman. Statistical analysis of strategic interaction with unobserved player actions: Introducing a strategic probit with partial observability. *Political Analysis*, 23(3):429–448, 2015.

A. K. Nikoloulopoulos. On the estimation of normal copula discrete regression models using the continuous extension and simulated likelihood. *Journal of Statistical Planning and Inference*, 143(11):1923–1937, 2013.

A. K. Nikoloulopoulos and D. Karlis. Regression in a copula model for bivariate count data. *Journal of Applied Statistics*, 37(9):1555–1568, 2010.

J. Nocedal and S. J. Wright. *Numerical Optimization*. Springer Series in Operations Research, 2006.

A. J. Oswald. Happiness and economic performance. *The Economic Journal*, 107(445): 1815–1831, 1997.

M. Pitt, D. Chan, and R. Kohn. Efficient Bayesian inference for Gaussian copula regression models. *Biometrika*, 93(3):537–554, 2006.

D. J. Poirier. Partial observability in bivariate probit models. *Journal of Econometrics*, 12 (2):209–217, 1980.

R. Radice, G. Marra, and M. Wojtyś. Copula regression spline models for binary outcomes. *Statistics and Computing*, 26(5):981–995, 2016.

N. Reid. A conversation with Sir David Cox. *Statistical Science*, 9(3):439–455, 1994.

P. Royston and P. C. Lambert. *Flexible Parametric Survival Analysis Using Stata: Beyond the Cox Model*. First edition. Stata Press, 2011.

P. H. C. Sant'Anna. Nonparametric tests for treatment effect heterogeneity with duration outcomes. *Journal of Business & Economic Statistics*, 39(3):816–832, 2021.

G. E. Schwarz. Estimating the dimension of a model. *The Annals of Statistics*, 6(2):461–464, 1978.

P. Shi and E. A. Valdez. Multivariate negative binomial models for insurance claim counts. *Insurance: Mathematics and Economics*, 55(9):18–29, 2014.

H. Shono. Application of the Tweedie distribution to zero-catch data in CPUE analysis. *Fisheries Research*, 93(1–2):154–162, 2008.

J. Siddique, M. J. Daniels, G. Inan, S. Battalio, B. Spring, and D. Hedeker. Joint modeling the frequency and duration of accelerometer-measured physical activity from a lifestyle intervention trial. *Statistics in Medicine*, 42(28):5100–5112, 2023.

A. Silva, S. J. Rothstein, P. D. McNicholas, and S. Subedi. A multivariate Poisson-log normal mixture model for clustering transcriptome sequencing data. *BMC Bioinformatics*, 20(1):394, 2019.

E. Solomon-Moore, R. Salway, L. Emm-Collison, J. L. Thompson, S. J. Sebire, D. A. Lawlor, and R. Jago. Associations of body mass index, physical activity and sedentary time with blood pressure in primary school children from South-West England: A prospective study. *PLoS ONE*, 15(4):e0232333, 2020.

M. Spiess. Estimation of a two-equation panel model with mixed continuous and ordered categorical outcomes and missing data. *Journal of the Royal Statistical Society Series C*, 55(4):525–538, 2006.

M. D. Stasinopoulos, R. A. Rigby, G. Z. Heller, V. Voudouris, and F. De Bastiani. *Flexible Regression and Smoothing Using GAMLSS in R*. Chapman & Hall/CRC, 2017.

M. D. Stasinopoulos, T. Kneib, N. Klein, A. Mayr, and G. Z. Heller. *Generalized Additive Models for Location, Scale and Shape: A Distributional Regression Approach, with Applications*. Cambridge University Press, 2024.

F. Tanser, V. Hosegood, T. Bärnighausen, K. Herbst, M. Nyirenda, W. Muhwava, C. Newell, J. Viljoen, T. Mutevedzi, and M. L. Newell. Cohort profile: Africa Centre Demographic Information system (ACDIS) and population-based HIV survey. *International Journal of Epidemiology*, 37(5):956–962, 2007.

M. Teimourian, T. Baghfalaki, M. Ganjali, and D. Berridge. Joint modeling of mixed skewed continuous and ordinal longitudinal responses: A Bayesian approach. *Journal of Applied Statistics*, 42(10):2233–2256, 2015.

P. Trivedi and D. Zimmer. *Copula Modeling: An Introduction for Practitioners*. Foundations and Trends in Econometrics, 2007.

H. van der Wurp, A. Groll, T. Kneib, G. Marra, and R. Radice. Generalised joint regression for count data: A penalty extension for competitive settings. *Statistics and Computing*, 30 (5):1419–1432, 2020.

Q. H. Vuong. Likelihood ratio tests for model selection and non-nested hypotheses. *Econometrica*, 57(2):307–333, 1989.

A. A. Weiss. A bivariate ordered probit model with truncation: Helmet use and motorcycle injuries. *Journal of the Royal Statistical Society Series C*, 42(3):487–499, 1993.

S. N. Wood. *Generalized Additive Models: An Introduction With R*. Second edition. Chapman & Hall/CRC, 2017.

S. A. Woodbury and R. G. Spiegelman. Bonuses to workers and employers to reduce unemployment: Randomized trials in illinois. *The American Economic Review*, 77(4): 513–530, 1987.

L. Yang. Diagnostics for regression models with semicontinuous outcomes. *Biometrics*, 80 (1):ujae007, 2024.

L. Yang, E. W. Frees, and Z. Zhang. Nonparametric estimation of copula regression models with discrete outcomes. *Journal of the American Statistical Association*, 115(530):707–720, 2020.

G. Yin and Y. Yuan. Bayesian dose finding in oncology for drug combinations by copula regression. *Journal of the Royal Statistical Society Series C*, 58(2):211–224, 2009.

N. Younes and J. Lachin. Link-based models for survival data with interval and continuous time censoring. *Biometrics*, 53(4):1199–1211, 1997.

H. Zhu and M. C. Wang. Analysing bivariate survival data with interval sampling and application to cancer epidemiology. *Biometrika*, 99(2):345–361, 2012.

Index

Note: Page numbers in **bold** and *italic* refer to tables and figures, respectively.

For Product Safety Concerns and Information please contact our EU
representative GPSR@taylorandfrancis.com
Taylor & Francis Verlag GmbH, Kaufingerstraße 24, 80331 München, Germany